The **Vegetative State**

The strange and harrowing sight of a person being awake but unaware with no evidence of a working mind – characteristics of the vegetative state – provokes intense debate and raises profound questions for health professionals, ethicists, philosophers and lawyers. This unique account by an unrivalled expert in the field, who himself collaborated in coining the term 'persistent vegetative state', surveys the medical, ethical and legal issues that surround this controversial topic. The medical definition and criteria for diagnosis are discussed, as are its frequency and causes, and possible outcomes. These range from some recovery to death, with some surviving indefinitely in a vegetative state, which some people believe is a fate worse than death. Ethical arguments discussed include the conflict between sanctity of life and respect for the autonomy and best interests of the victim, and between killing and letting die. Legal issues are explored with details of landmark court cases from the USA, Britain and elsewhere. This well-informed and carefully constructed account will be a benchmark for medical specialists, ethicists, lawyers and philosophers.

Bryan Jennett has had a long and distinguished career with unrivalled insight into the vegetative state. As Professor of Neurosurgery at the University of Glasgow his research was instrumental in defining the condition, and in coining the term 'persistent vegetative state'. Since then he has continued to write extensively on this subject, to lecture widely around the world, and has been an expert witness in a number of key court cases.

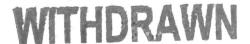

The **Vegetative State**

Medical facts, ethical and legal dilemmas

Bryan Jennett

University of Glasgow, Scotland

Foreword by Fred Plum

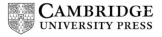
CAMBRIDGE
UNIVERSITY PRESS

PUBLISHED BY THE PRESS SYNDICATE OF THE UNIVERSITY OF CAMBRIDGE
The Pitt Building, Trumpington Street, Cambridge, United Kingdom

CAMBRIDGE UNIVERSITY PRESS
The Edinburgh Building, Cambridge CB2 2RU, UK
40 West 20th Street, New York, NY 10011–4211, USA
477 Williamstown Road, Port Melbourne, VIC 3207, Australia
Ruiz de Alarcón 13, 28014 Madrid, Spain
Dock House, The Waterfront, Cape Town 8001, South Africa

http://www.cambridge.org

First published 2002
Reprinted 2003

Printed in the United Kingdom at the University Press, Cambridge

Typeface Minion 10.5/13pt   *System* Poltype® [v N]

A catalogue record for this book is available from the British Library

Library of Congress Cataloguing in Publication data

Jennett, Bryan.
The vegetative state: medical facts, ethical and legal dilemmas / Bryan Jennett.
    p.   cm.
Includes bibliographical references and index.
ISBN 0 521 44158 7
1. Persistent vegetative state.   I. Title.
RB150.C6 J46 2002
616.8'49–dc21   2001037373

ISBN 0 521 44158 7 paperback

Contents

Foreword   vii
Preface   ix
Acknowledgements   xi
An appeal to doctors   xii
Traumatic decortication   xiii
List of abbreviations   xiv

1   A syndrome in search of a name   1

2   Diagnosis   7

3   Epidemiology   33

4   Pathology of the brain damage   51

5   Prognosis for recovery and survival   57

6   Attitudes to the permanent vegetative state   73

7   Medical management   87

8   Ethical issues   97

9   Legal issues in the United States   127

10 Legal issues in Britain   147

11 Legal issues in other countries   173

12 Details of some landmark cases   187

Epilogue   221
Index   223

Foreword

Professor Bryan Jennett has led the world in understanding the devastating unconscious condition termed the vegetative state. New forms of bedside, physiologically oriented ventilators and other supportive devices for maintaining lives around the world started to develop in the late 1940s. Much of this technology was grouped in critical poliomyelitis centres, but after 1955, as polio epidemics became prevented by vaccination, only a few institutions world wide developed critical-care programmes that received all kinds of severely ill patients. These centres required doctors specially trained to handle both medical and surgical crises, but unfortunately it took some years for small hospitals to understand the importance of transferring critically ill patients rapidly to such centers in large teaching hospitals. At this point, in the late 1960s, Professor Jennett and his associates were developing and testing their own, now famous, Glasgow Coma Scale (GCS) for traumatic brain injury. Their first goal was to estimate the acute findings of the GCS with the patients' current symptoms and signs. They then compared the initial scale against the patients' ultimate outcomes. The quality of outcome in patients who were immediately referred to the Glasgow University Hospitals was greatly better than those who remained to be treated in smaller hospitals. It was an astonishing success. But even with the best treatment some severely ill patients whose lives had been saved were left with severe permanent brain damage.

Knowing of this work I had the rewarding opportunity of discussing with Professor Jennett, both in New York and Glasgow, the significance of GCS scores and outcomes and how they could be modified to evaluate severe medical illnesses and medically related catastrophic accidents. Following visits to Glasgow and other large UK hospitals, as well as some in the USA, we gained support from the US National Institutes of Health (NIH) to study the prognosis of coma resulting from asystole, asphyxial stroke and other severe dysfunctional medical conditions, as well as from traumatic brain injury. During these fruitful years Professor Jennett and I coined the term 'the vegetative state', which has become rapidly understood by the medical profession.

As Professor Jennett emphasizes in this fine monograph, the judicial systems of both Britain and America relatively quickly came to understand the public's emotional and cost-conscious reaction to vegetative loved ones. Following the lead of American courts, British judges placed the responsibility of maintaining or withdrawing medical care for permanently vegetative patients in the courts. With the advantage of the general homogeneity of the British people, the judges in the UK have been able to review the law progressively and to agree individually with doctors and families how best to deal with such hopelessly unconscious patients. In the USA, there is a much greater heterogeneity in religion, in widely spread global ancestry, and even in currently spoken languages. This, together with different laws in different states, has made it more difficult to reach a national consensus on these matters.

As well as correlating a mass of medical information, Professor Jennett has presented us with a valuable dissertation on ethical issues, their specific qualities and their strong relationships with the law in many countries. The book is a treasure chest of the associations that exist between ethics, customs, language, homogeneity of population, and strong relationships to science and to religion.

We thank him for his sensibility and will read him many times over.

Fred Plum, MD

Preface

The life-sustaining technologies associated with resuscitation and intensive care make it possible now for many patients to survive an episode of acute brain damage so severe that it would previously have proved rapidly fatal. Some such rescued patients make a good recovery, some survive only briefly, whilst others are left with permanent brain damage of varying degrees. In its most severe form this damage leaves the patient without any normal function in the cerebral cortex, and therefore bereft of thought or perception. Although these patients have periods with their eyes open, and are thus apparently awake, they show no evidence of being aware of their surroundings or of having a working mind. They are said to be in a vegetative state. For some this is a temporary state that is followed by some degree of recovery, but others are left permanently vegetative and they can survive like this for many years if life-sustaining treatment and nursing care are provided.

In the 30 years since this state was first described it has provoked intense debate among health professionals, clinical scientists, moral philosophers and lawyers. It is the strange combination of being awake but unaware with no evidence of a working mind that is so disturbing and puzzling. When a patient is left permanently vegetative this is widely perceived to be an outcome of medical intervention that is worse than death. The controversial question then arises as to whether it is appropriate to prolong their lives indefinitely by further medical treatment. Many cases have come to court for judicial review of a decision to withdraw life-sustaining treatment, initially in the USA but recently also in Britain and elsewhere. Certain high profile cases have reached the highest courts – *Cruzan* in the US Supreme Court and *Bland* in the House of Lords. Several cases have provoked eager media interest. This has led to an unusual degree of public awareness of this condition and there are said to be over a thousand web sites devoted to it. The issue of how such patients should be treated is seen as having wider public policy implications, particularly in relation to the debate about euthanasia. As a result there have been position papers from doctors, moralists and lawyers in several countries about the dilemma posed by vegetative patients, and the attitudes of doctors towards them in different member States have been surveyed in a research project of the European Commission. However, the vegetative state is relatively uncommon, with few professionals and fewer of the public ever having encountered such a patient.

It therefore seemed timely to review what is known medically about the vegetative state and how prolonged survival in this state is viewed by doctors and others in society. The early chapters consider how its nomenclature has evolved, and review the extensive medical literature on how it is diagnosed, how often it occurs, the causes and nature of the underlying brain pathology, and the prospects for recovery and survival. Attitudes to the permanent vegetative state are considered next, and a brief account is given of its medical management. The later chapters deal with the ethical and legal issues that have arisen in various countries when deciding how to deal with permanently vegetative patients, with detailed accounts of some landmark cases that have reached the courts in several countries. The medical and legal reports and ethical commentaries on this subject are widely scattered in specialist journals. The opportunity has been taken to bring these together in order to provide an accessible source for professionals in the different relevant disciplines and interested members of the public, who wish to broaden their perspective.

Acknowledgements

Charlotte Boulnois and Alistair Shields of the Central Library, Southern General Hospital, Glasgow were most helpful and resourceful in obtaining articles from a range of journals far beyond their regular repertoire and I am most grateful to them. Professor Hume Adams kindly vetted the chapter on pathology for me. My secretary, Madeleine Younger, brought her usual consummate skills to initial drafts of this text.

I acknowledge permission to reproduce Dr Beernink's poem from the *Lancet*, Table 2.3 from the *Annals of Neurology*, Tables 2.8, 2.9 and 2.10 from the *Journal of Neurology, Neurosurgery & Psychiatry*, and Tables 3.17 and 3.18 from *Advances in Pediatrics*, John Wiley and Son.

An appeal to doctors

It adds fresh terror to traffic to know that an accident may make you an unconscious hulk lasting for years, a sorrow to any who love you, and a trouble to all concerned, wasting valuable nurses and resources. At best you could die in the end unconscious, at worst recover some degree of awareness and live indefinitely, deprived of all those powers which distinguish us from the lower animals. The ability to prolong life may be a curse instead of a blessing.

From a letter in the *Lancet* from a Cambridge University physicist.

Thompson GT. An appeal to doctors *Lancet* 1969; 2: 1353

Traumatic decortication

Always the blinds were pulled in your room where you waited,
Patient as a pupa, for a diaper change or a turn
Onto last week's bedsore. Your sightless eyes would burn
White in the dark while your soul crouched in the corner.

Monthly that winter your mother came and repeated
Her convictions that you, 'would soon be looking better',
And proudly numbered the gooks you'd killed before
The shrapnel buried you mind in Asia's mud.

For a year synthetic life had been pumped to your blood
Through dozens of tubes. Each day the residents
Were pleased to see your heart and lungs were clear –
Organs serving no intelligence.

Then one morning we found your BIRD[a] unplugged.
    The corner
Was empty. I opened the blinds. Spring was near.

[a](BIRD is a respirator)

From 'Ward Rounds', a book of poems about particular patients, by Dr K.D. Beernink, 1970.

Lowbury EJL Ward rounds. *Lancet* 1970; ii: 924

Abbreviations

AAN	American Academy of Neurology
ALERT	Against Legalized Euthanasia – Research and Teaching
AMA	American Medical Association
ANA	American Neurological Association
ANH	Artificial nutrition and hydration
BMA	British Medical Association
CBF	Cerebral blood flow
CPR	Cardiopulmonary resuscitation
CT	Computerized tomography
DA	District attorney
DAI	Diffuse axonal injury
DNR	Do not resuscitate
EEG	Electroencephalogram
MCS	Minimally conscious state
MP	Member of parliament
MRI	Magnetic resonance imaging
NHS	National Health Service
PEG	Percutaneous endoscopic gastrostomy
PET	Positron emission tomography
PMP	per million population
PVS	Persistent or permanent vegetative state (in legal chapters, always denotes permanent)
VS	Vegetative state

A syndrome in search of a name

When Jennett and Plum in 1972 coined the term persistent vegetative state, in a *Lancet* paper subtitled 'A syndrome in search of a name' (1), they were neither the first to describe this condition nor the first to propose a name. In 1899, Rosenblath had reported a 15-year-old tightrope walker who after two weeks in coma following a fall from his wire recovered 'to become strangely awake'; he died after 8 months being tube fed in this state (2). In 1940, a German psychiatrist Kretschmer proposed the term **the apallic syndrome** to describe patients who were awake but unresponsive (3). As examples he described a case with a gunshot wound of both cerebral hemispheres and one of panencephalitis subacuta, thereby indicating that this state could result from either acute or chronic progressive brain damage. Although several authors in continental Europe have used this term (4) it has never caught on in English-speaking countries.

In 1952 an American neurosurgeon commented that when brain damage deprived patients of the intuitive and protective functions necessary for survival they rarely lived more than 2–3 weeks (5). However, he went on to describe five patients who had survived for months with periods of wakefulness without ever being aware, but he did not suggest a name for this state. In 1956, Strich reported the pathological findings in five cases from the Oxford Neurosurgical Unit who had what she called **severe traumatic dementia** (6). She commented on the similarity between the severe white matter degeneration that she found and that previously reported by Rosenblath in his case. Since then others have used the term **post-traumatic dementia** or **encephalopathy**, but these terms have never acquired the strict definition now associated with the vegetative state. In fact, in her expanded series of 20 such patients examined pathologically, Strich noted that several had spoken a few words and some had even obeyed commands during the stage of partial recovery before they died (7). Similarly, those using the apallic label frequently referred to partial or incomplete forms of the syndrome (8). By contrast, Jennett and Plum recommended an absolute distinction between patients who did not make any consistently understandable response to those around them, whether by word or by gesture, and those who never did. The former should be regarded as very severely disabled and not as in a lesser degree of the vegetative state. Recently the terms **minimally responsive state** (9) or **minimally conscious state** (10) have emerged to describe those patients who have regained very limited conscious responses (p. 23).

The terms **permanent, irreversible** or **prolonged coma** or **unconsciousness** have been used at various times to describe vegetative patients, and still sometimes appear in articles (or headlines) by journalists. However, physicians now generally accept that **coma** should be confined to describing patients whose eyes are continuously closed and who cannot be aroused to a wakeful state. Of course many patients in a vegetative state following an acute insult will have been in coma for some time before regaining wakefulness, although some nontraumatic cases may become vegetative after only a day or so in coma. This is because there has been no element of widespread temporary depression of the reticular activating system that is a consistent feature of severe head injury. **Unconsciousness** is taken to imply lack of awareness of the self or the environment. The President's Commission in 1983 accepted several types of patient as having permanent loss of consciousness (11). These included those in a vegetative state (duration undefined), those in coma from acute brain damage till death, in coma from untreatable mass lesions or in the end stage of degenerative conditions such as Alzheimer's disease, and infants with anencephaly. Both patients in coma and those in a vegetative state are unconscious but this term fails to distinguish between the two because it does not acknowledge that arousal and awareness can be independently affected. Some have suggested that vegetative patients be described as having prolonged **post-traumatic unawareness** (12) or **postcomatose unawareness** (13).

These patients have sometimes been described as in a **decerebrate** or **decorticate state**. These terms are most often used to describe types of motor dysfunction rather than the mental state implied by the term vegetative. Moreover, these terms tend to imply structural lesions that do not correspond to the pathological findings in all vegetative patients. Physiologists commonly use decerebration to describe the state of animals after upper brain stem transection and this would be anatomically misleading when applied to patients in the vegetative state.

Coma vigile was sometimes used in the older French literature to describe some patients with severe typhus and typhoid fever, and although it is neatly descriptive of one aspect of the vegetative state it does not adequately encompass the syndrome as a whole (14).

Akinetic mutism was coined by Cairns et al. in 1941 (15) to describe the intermittent depression of consciousness observed in an adolescent with a brain tumour (craniopharyngioma). Her condition was one of silent immobility, with the eyes open and apparently attentive, and 'giving the promise of speech' – indeed she sometimes did whisper in monosyllables. Her state was three times reversed by aspirating fluid from the tumour. A subsequent review by Skultety (16) found this term to be used rather loosely to describe reversible disorders of responsiveness in which akinesis and mutism did not always go together – some patients spoke or used sign language. Nor were the limbs in the spastic posture associated with the vegetative state. He ascribed it to functional depression of critical amounts of the afferent or efferent systems, or of the activating reticular formation. Again, the term is descriptive of only part of the behaviour of vegetative patients and it is not an acceptable synonym.

Neocortical necrosis is a pathological term that applies only to the subset of vegetative patients who have suffered anoxic or hypoglycaemic damage resulting in loss of cortical neurones. The term **cognitive death** has some attraction in that it invites comparison with, but a distinction from, brain death, but the term death implies irreversibility.

The phrase **pie vegetative** was used by Arnaud et al. in 1963 to describe some survivors of head injury (17), and **vegetative survival** was one outcome category for severe head injuries reported by the Finnish neurosurgeons Vapalahti and Troupp in 1971 (18), but their condition was not clearly defined. The term persistent vegetative state (PVS) came the following year, with arguments that it was preferable to all previous names (1). Its acceptance into medical terminology in many countries probably owes much to its being one of the four categories of survival in the Glasgow Outcome Scale proposed by Jennett and Bond in 1975 (19). This scale has been widely adopted by neurosurgeons and neurologists for reporting the outcome in survivors of either traumatic or nontraumatic coma.

Persistent vegetative state (PVS) was recommended as the term of choice in the 1993 report of the American Neurological Association (20) and in the 1994 statement of the Multi-Society Task Force (21), and it has been widely adopted also by philosophers, lawyers and others outside medicine. As Jennett and Plum (1) stated, the word vegetative itself is not obscure. **To**

vegetate is defined in the Oxford English dictionary as 'to live a merely physical life, devoid of intellectual activity or social intercourse (1740)', and **vegetative** is used to describe 'an organic body capable of growth and development but devoid of sensation and thought (1764)'. It suggests even to the layman a limited and primitive responsiveness to external stimuli, whilst it reminds the doctor that there is relative preservation of autonomic regulation of the internal milieu of the body.

In seeking a name for this syndrome we wished to have one that did not presume a particular anatomical abnormality or pathological lesion because these vary considerably from case to case and can seldom be known with certainty at the bedside. A term that described behaviour seemed appropriate as the essence of the definition is observed behaviour, and is independent of special investigations that may not always be available, and that in any event do not show consistent abnormalities in vegetative patients (pp. 25–8). As our intention was to provide a term that would facilitate communication about this state between doctors and the patient's relatives, moralists and lawyers it seemed advantageous to have one that avoided medical jargon. Moreover such a broad descriptive term, indicating only absence of observed cognitive function, invited further clinical and pathological investigations rather than giving the impression of a problem already fully understood.

In recent years there has, however, been increasing concern about the ambiguity of the 'persistent' component of this term because it may seem to suggest irreversibility, although Jennett and Plum had made it clear that this should not be implied. Recovery of varying degrees after weeks and sometimes months in a vegetative state is now widely recognized, but confusion is evident in occasional statements that the diagnosis of PVS cannot be made until a year after an acute brain insult. This is to confuse diagnosis with prognosis. There is no doubt that the label PVS in the first few weeks after a brain insult can result in suboptimal rehabilitation efforts at a stage when active treatment is important, because recovery is still possible. For this reason expert groups in the US and Europe have suggested using only the terms 'vegetative state' and 'permanent vegetative state' (22,23,24,25). Indeed, the authoritative code of practice published by the Royal College of Physicians of London in 1996 was titled 'The permanent vegetative state' (25). This recommended using 'the vegetative state' for the condition soon after the insult, the 'continuing vegetative state' when it had lasted for more than four weeks and 'permanent vegetative state' when it was considered to have become irreversible (by agreed criteria). In the rest of this book PVS will be used only to refer to the permanent vegetative state, but it must be accepted that this abbreviation is still widely used to mean persistent rather than permanent.

Some commentators, including the Pro-Life Committee of Catholic Bishops in the US (26), have expressed concern that the word vegetative can suggest that the patient is a vegetable and therefore subhuman, and they have urged the medical profession to seek a less discriminatory and demeaning alternative. Several physicians share this concern and some US and UK experts have suggested as an alternative 'the wakeful unconscious state' (13). They did so without much confidence that the term vegetative state was likely to be replaced because it is now so widely used by many different disciplines.

REFERENCES

1 Jennett B, Plum F. Persistent vegetative state after brain damage. A syndrome in search of a name. *Lancet* 1972; 1: 734–7

2 Rosenblath W. Uber einen bemerkenswerten Fall von Hirnerschutterung. *Dtsch Arch Klin Med* 1899; 64: 406–24

3 Kretschmer E. Das apallische syndrom. *Z Gesante Neurol Psychiatr, Berlin* 1940; 169: 576–9

4 Ore GD, Gerstenbrand F, Lucking CH. *The Apallic Syndrome*. Berlin: Springer-Verlag, 1977

5 French JD. Brain lesions associated with prolonged unconsciousness. *Arch Neurol Psychiatry* 1952; 68: 727–40

6 Strich SJ. Diffuse degeneration of cerebral white matter and severe dementia following head injury. *J Neurol Neurosurg Psychiatry* 1956; 19: 163–85

7 Strich SJ. Shearing of nerve fibres as a cause of brain damage due to head injury. *Lancet* 1961; 2: 444–8

8 Gerstenbrand F. *Das traumatische apallische syndrom*. Vienna and New York: Springer 1967

9 Giacino JT, Zasler ND. Outcome following severe brain injury. The comatose, vegetative and minimally responsive patient. *J Head Trauma Rehabil* 1995; 10: 40–56

10 Giacino J, Ashwal S, Childs N et al. The minimally conscious state: definition and diagnostic criteria. *Neurology* 2001; 57: in press

11 President's Commission for the Study of Ethical Problems in Medicine. *Deciding to*

forego life-sustaining treatment. Washington DC: US Government Printing Office, 1983

12 Sazbon L, Groswasser Z. Outcome in 134 patients with prolonged post-traumatic unawareness. Part 1: Parameters determining late recovery of consciousness. *J Neurosurg* 1990; 72: 75–80

13 Sazbon L, Groswasser Z. Prolonged coma, vegetative state, post-comatose unawareness: semantics or better understandings? *Brain Injury* 1995; 5: 1–2

14 Alajouanine T. Les altérations des états de conscience causes par les désordres neurologiques. *Acta Med Belgium* 1957; 2: 19–41

15 Cairns H, Oldfield RC, Pennybacker JB et al. Akinetic mutism with an epidermoid cyst of the third ventricle. *Brain* 1941; 64: 273–90

16 Skultety FM. Clinical and experimental aspects of akinetic mutism. *Arch Neurol* 1968; 17: 1–148

17 Arnaud M, Vigouroux R, Vigouroux M. États frontiers entre la vie et la mort en neuro-traumatologie. *Neurochirurgia (Stuttg)* 1963; 6: 1–21

18 Vapalahti M, Troupp H. Prognosis for patients with severe head injuries. *BMJ* 1971; iii: 404–7

19 Jennett B, Bond M. Assessment of outcome after severe brain damage. A practical scale. *Lancet* 1975; 1: 480–84

20 American Neurological Association Committee on Ethical Affairs. Persistent vegetative state. *Ann Neurol* 1993; 33: 386–90

21 The Multi-Society Task Force on the Persistent Vegetative State. Statement on medical aspects of the persistent vegetative state. *N Engl J Med* 1994; 330: 1499–508

22 American Congress of Rehabilitation Medicine. Recommendations for use of uniform nomenclature pertinent to patients with severe alterations of consciousness. *Arch Phys Med Rehabil* 1995; 76: 205–9

23 Zasler ND. Nomenclature: evolving trends. *NeuroRehabilitation* 1996; 6: 3–8

24 Health Council of the Netherlands Committee on Vegetative State. *Patients in a vegetative state.* The Hague, Health Council of the Netherlands, 1994

25 Royal College of Physicians Working Group. The permanent vegetative state. *J R Coll Physicians Lond* 1996; 30: 119–21

26 Committee for Pro-Life Activities of the National Conference of Catholic Bishops. Nutrition and hydration: moral and pastoral reflections. *Issues Law Med* 1992; 8: 387–406

2

Diagnosis

The definition of the vegetative state and the description of its features have evolved over the years as individuals have reported surveys of patients and as various medical organizations have produced consensus statements. Criteria used for two widely quoted Japanese epidemiological surveys in the late 1970s now seem very imprecise (Tables 2.1 and 2.2), but they may have lost something in translation. However, it is clear that the definition of Sato et al. (2) allowed inclusion of patients who could obey some commands and who would therefore have been excluded by later definitions. The responses of 250 child neurologists (3) who were asked in 1991 to comment on the relative importance of ten features that had been proposed as an operational definition of vegetative state by Nelson and Bernat (4) showed a marked lack of consensus (Table 2.3). An estimate of the prevalence of the vegetative state in children in California in 1991 was based on a survey of State residents registered as developmentally disabled (5). To identify residents who might be considered to be in a vegetative state 15 items were selected from the adaptive behavioural section of the Client Development Evaluation Report form (Table 2.4). However, this form had been devised for other purposes and there must be some doubt as to how accurately this group of items corresponds with more formal definitions of the vegetative state that have emerged since then.

A committee of the American Neurological Association (ANA) (6) published a set of diagnostic criteria in 1993 (Table 2.5). Then came the 1994 report from The Multi-Society Task Force on PVS (7), which included representatives from five American professional bodies – the Academy of Neurology, the Neurological Association, the Association of Neurological Surgeons, the Academy of Pediatrics and the Child Neurology Society. The report included a list of criteria (Table 2.6), which represented codified elaborations of the more descriptive accounts given by Jennett and Plum in 1972 (8), by the American Academy of Neurology

Table 2.1. Epidemiological survey in Japan 1977

Arbitrary criteria for study

1. Defect of verbal and behavioural communication
2. Loss of expression of intention
3. Absence, or at least reduction, of emotional expression
4. Urinary and faecal incontinence
5. Complete loss of self-supportability

Higashi et al. (1).

Table 2.2. Epidemiological survey in Japan 1978

1. Unable to move by himself
2. Able to vocalize but unable to make any meaningful speech
3. Can barely respond to such a simple order as 'open your eyes', 'squeeze my hand', etc. but no further communication is possible
4. Eyes can follow an object but cannot recognize it
5. Unable to take a meal by himself
6. Be in a state of rectal and urinary incontinence

Based on promulgation of Japanese Neurosurgical Society, Sato et al. (2).

(AAN) in 1989 (9) and by the American Medical Association (AMA) in 1990 (10). The Quality Standards Subcommittee of the American Academy of Neurology (11) subsequently endorsed the Task Force criteria, and they have become the benchmark for American practice. In 1996, the Royal College of Physicians of London produced a statement (12) in response to a request from a parliamentary committee set up after the *Bland* case (p. 154), and this included diagnostic criteria (Table 2.7). It is to be hoped that these authoritative declarations will limit the variation in definition that was evident in some early reports.

Features of the vegetative state

What characterizes the vegetative state is the combination of periods of wakeful eye opening without any evidence of a working mind either receiving or projecting information, a dissociation between arousal and

Table 2.3. Responses of 250 child neurologists to commonly used features of PVS (% of respondents)

	Apply	Supportive	Necessary
Wakefulness without awareness	95	16	84
Eyes-open unconsciousness	94	33	67
No 'voluntary' action or behaviour	91	23	77
No 'cognitive' response	90	22	78
No 'voluntary' language	84	29	71
No commands followed	83	22	78
No sustained eye tracking	83	47	53
Intact brain stem reflexes, sleep/wake cycles	75	53	47
Breathing intact, chewing and swallowing impaired	75	65	35
Bowel and bladder incontinence	53	53	47

From Ashwal et al. (3).

awareness. Following acute insults the eyes open spontaneously after a period that varies according to the mechanism of the brain insult. Head injury involves a concussive effect on the brain-stem reticular formation that takes time to recover, and it is usually 2–3 weeks, sometimes as long as 12 weeks, before the eyes open and coma ends. After nontraumatic coma, when there is no concussion, the eyes open much sooner, in more than half the patients in the first week, in some within 24 hours of the insult (13). However, in Higashi's series of 110 cases who had all been vegetative for at least 3 months, half of them for more than a year, 14% still had their eyes closed at this time and this was still so for 4% at follow-up 3 years later (1). It is exceptionally rare for true coma to be so prolonged; it never lasted more than a month in a large series of survivors of nontraumatic coma (13). It may, however, occur with a lesion in the posterior hypothalamus (14). Another possible explanation for failure of the eyes to open for a long period after head injury is that focal damage has produced bilateral third nerve lesions resulting in ptosis (paralysis of the muscle that opens the eyelids). Once the eyes do open, patients in a vegetative state have prolonged periods of being awake, alternating with sleep (from which they can be roused by vigorous stimulation). Whether this periodicity reflects normal diurnal rhythm is difficult to assess, because such patients are usually

Table 2.4. Items from Client Development Evaluation Report used to define vegetative patients in survey of disabled in California

1. Rolling and sitting: does not lift head when on stomach; no rolling or sitting
2. Hand use: no functional hand use
3. Arm use: no functional arm use
4. Eating: does not feed self, must be fed completely
5. Level of bladder control: no control
6. Level of bowel control: no control
7. One-to-one interaction with peers: does not enter into interaction
8. Auditory perception: does not react to sounds
9. Visual perception: does not explore visually; includes continuous staring
10. Associating time with events and actions: does not associate events and actions with time
11. Word usage: no use of words
12. Expressive nonverbal communication: no expressive nonverbal communication
13. Receptive nonverbal communication: does not demonstrate understanding of gestures (tactile or visual) or facial expressions
14. Receptive language: does not understand speech
15. Expressive language: makes no sound

From Ashwal et al. (5).

in continual light and frequently stimulated, as part of their active nursing care.

Whilst eye opening is a positive and uncontroversial feature of the vegetative state, the crux of the rest of the definition is essentially negative – the lack of any evidence of awareness, by meaningful responses or activity. However, the wide range of reflex responsiveness in vegetative patients, and the tendency for this to become more marked as time passes in most patients, can give rise to some such activity being interpreted as evidence of returning consciousness. Because some vegetative patients do recover consciousness it is important to recognize when that boundary is reached and the patient can be declared no longer vegetative but in a minimally conscious state (p. 24) or even better than that. What is clear is that some patients can regain a wide repertoire of reflex responsiveness without going on to recover any evidence of awareness when followed for months or years, whilst some 'recovered' patients may not progress beyond a state of minimal consciousness. The only detailed report of the frequency of

Table 2.5. American Neurological Association Committee on Ethical Affairs 1993

The following criteria should be met

1. The patient displays no evidence of awareness of self or surroundings. Reflex or spontaneous eye opening may occur.
2. No communication between the examiner and the patient, auditory or written, that is meaningful and consistent can be established. Target stimuli are not usually followed visually, although visual tracking can occasionally occur. There is no emotional response by the patient to verbal input.
3. There is no comprehensible speech or mouthing of words.
4. Smiling, frowning, and crying may occur occasionally but are inconsistently related to any apparent stimulus.
5. Sleep–wake cycles are present.
6. Brain-stem and spinal reflex activity is variable. Primitive reflexes such as sucking, rooting, chewing and swallowing may be preserved. Pupillary reactivity to light, oculocephalic reflexes, grasp reflexes and tendon reflexes may be present.
7. The presence of voluntary movements or behaviour, no matter how rudimentary, is a sign of cognition and is incompatible with the diagnosis of PVS. There is no motor activity suggesting learned behaviour and no mimicry. Rudimentary movements (such as withdrawal or posturing) may be seen with noxious or disagreeable stimuli.
8. Blood pressure control and cardiorespiratory functions usually are intact. Incontinence of bladder and bowel is present.

From ANA report (6).

occurrence of a wide range of responses and behaviours in a series of vegetative patients was that of Higashi et al. (1) (Tables 2.8, 2.9 and 2.10), but these patients might not all have been vegetative by recent definitions. Beyond this there are only reports of the frequency of some behaviours in occasional series and the generalizations in the consensus statements of expert groups.

Much of the debate about diagnosis turns on what behaviours reflect cortical activity, and whether fragments of activity in the cortex necessarily indicates awareness – lack of which is the crux of the diagnosis of the vegetative state. It seems clear that cortical integrity is not required for sudden light or sound to stimulate a brief orienting reflex with the eyes blinking and the head and eyes turning briefly towards a strong auditory or visual stimulus. This, or even touching, may produce a general startle

Table 2.6. Statement of the Multi-Society Task Force 1994

Definition
The vegetative state is a condition of complete unawareness of the self and the environment accompanied by sleep–wake cycles with either complete or partial preservation of hypothalamic and brain stem autonomic functions.

Criteria
No evidence of awareness of themselves or their environment; they are incapable of interacting with others.

No evidence of sustained reproducible, purposeful or voluntary behavioural responses to visual, auditory, tactile or noxious stimuli.

No evidence of language comprehension or expression.

Intermittent wakefulness –sleep–wake cycles.

Sufficiently preserved hypothalamic and autonomic functions to survive. Bowel and bladder incontinence.

Variably preserved cranial nerve reflexes (pupillary, oculocephalic, corneal, vestibulo-ocular, gag), and spinal reflexes.

From Task Force Report (7).

reaction involving a jerk of the limbs – startle myoclonus. In vegetative patients these responses do not habituate as they would in a person with a higher level of responsiveness in whom repeating the stimulus produces less and less response. The same goes for blinking in response to tapping the bridge of the nose. Blinking may also occur from a corneal reflex to the movement of air as a hand rapidly approaches the eyes, making it difficult to distinguish from a purely visual threat. Some authorities consider lack of response to a visual threat as one criterion of the vegetative state, whilst others accept that some vegetative patients do respond. It is a matter of debate whether blink to threat indicates a limited cortical activity or can represent processing at a subcortical level. In any event, response to visual threat is not *per se* evidence of awareness.

The open eyes commonly show roving movements which may be dys-conjugate. Brief fixation on to, and following of, an object can occur. Relatives frequently assert that the patient looks at them and claim to see recognition in their eyes, but this alone cannot be accepted as evidence that

Table 2.7. Royal College of Physicians of London 1996

Three clinical criteria all to be fulfilled

1. No evidence of awareness of self or environment. No volitional response to visual, auditory, tactile or noxious stimuli. No evidence of language comprehension or expression.
2. Cycles of eye closure and opening simulating sleep and waking.
3. Sufficiently preserved hypothalamic and brain stem function to maintain respiration and circulation.

Other clinical features

1. Incontinence of bladder and bowel. Spontaneous blinking and usually retained pupillary and corneal responses. Conjugate or dysconjugate tonic response to ice-water caloric testing.
2. No nystagmus to caloric testing. No visual fixation, tracking of moving objects with eyes or response to menace.
3. May be occasional movements of head and eyes towards sound or movement, and of trunk and limbs in purposeless way. May have startle myoclonus. May smile; may grimace to pain. May have roving eye movements.

From Royal College of Physicians Working Group (12).

a patient is not vegetative. The AMA has declared that vegetative patients do not consistently follow moving objects, whilst the ANA allows that visual tracking can **occasionally** occur. The Task Force noted that sustained visual pursuit is lacking in **most** patients.

In Higashi's series, eye following occurred in a third of patients and, curiously, was more common earlier rather than later in the time course of the vegetative state (Table 2.8). Because consistent and sustained visual pursuit is usually one of the first observable signs of recovery in patients who go on to regain consciousness, some consider that patients who show this phenomenon are no longer vegetative. However, there is no doubt that occasional patients do regain sustained visual pursuit, but over a further period of months or years develop no other behavioural evidence of consciousness. In one study only 20% of 55 vegetative patients had visual tracking compared with 82% of 49 in a minimally conscious state (15). An International Working Party in 1996 concluded that visual tracking could not be considered in isolation as evidence of whether a patient is vegetative or not (16). It seems best to adopt the Task Force conclusion: 'One should

Table 2.8. Reactivity and behavioural responses of vegetative patients

	Percentage of n		
	June 1973 ($n = 110$)	June 1974 ($n = 64$)	June 1976 ($n = 38$)
Blinking	90.7	88.3	100.0
Sleep–wake rhythm	86	93.5	94.7
Response to painful stimuli	84.4	90.2	81.6
Spontaneous eye movement	75.0	83.1	81.6
Yawning	73.8	82.0	76.3
Response to auditory stimuli	57.5	60.7	52.6
Swallowing	50.5	57.4	81.6
Chewing	46.2	57.6	31.2
Eye-following movement	42.7	32.7	31.4
Emotional expression	30.9	41.0	47.4

At initial survey in June 1973 duration of PVS was 49% for > 1 year, 33% for 3–6 months.
From Higashi et al. (1) with permission.

be extremely cautious in making a diagnosis of the vegetative state when there is any degree of sustained visual pursuit, consistent and reproducible visual fixation, or response to threatening gestures' (1).

The Royal College of Physicians criteria have caused some confusion in regard to eye signs. The request had been to draw up criteria for the diagnosis of the vegetative state similar to the UK criteria for brain death. The latter were based on establishing that there was no residual function in the brain stem and this led the College to propose criteria for the vegetative state that set out to show no sign of cortical function rather than lack of awareness (Table 2.7). In several cases since then, the English courts have chosen to accept expert opinion that particular patients were unaware and therefore vegetative although one or more of the eye responses listed by the College under 'other criteria' were still active (pp. 161–2).

The limbs are usually spastic and they may move in a nonpurposeful way and there may be groping movements. A grasp reflex may be set off by contact with bedclothes, the nasogastric tube or the hand of an observer and these may be misinterpreted as indicating voluntary movements or

Table 2.9. Neurological findings in vegetative patients

Finding	Percentage of n		
	June 1973 ($n=110$)	June 1974 ($n=64$)	June 1976 ($n=38$)
Aniscoria	21.2	22.4	14.7
Light reflex	73.7	64.4	78.4
Ciliospinal reflex	37.7	25.0	47.2
Optic nerve atrophy	39.0	34.7	54.8
Ciliary reflex	91.6	96.7	97.3
Abdominal reflex	10.0	28.2	45.5
Deep tendon reflexes			
Upper extremities			
Diminished	23.0	15.3	27.0
Exaggerated	31.0	39.0	48.6
Lower extremities			
Diminished	51.5	59.3	36.1
Exaggerated	30.7	23.7	38.9
Pyramidal tract signs	60.0	55.7	58.3
Primitive reflexes			
Snout	34.7	48.3	69.4
Grasping	19.4	19.7	22.9
Tonic neck	6.5	5.4	3.1

From Higashi et al. (1) with permission.

meaningful responses, especially by relatives seeking evidence for recovery. However, careful observation reveals no consistent movements that are voluntary or learned, or a response to command or mimicry. In Higashi's series (Table 2.10), a variety of motor patterns were seen which could be regarded as reflecting the patchy distribution of the brain damage found at autopsy in many cases (pp. 52–3). Most patients show some response to painful stimuli. A stimulated limb may withdraw or there may be a generalized movement of all four limbs, sometimes accompanied by facial grimacing and perhaps a groan. There may also be a rise in respiratory and pulse rates and in blood pressure. It is generally held that these responses are all at reflex level and do not indicate that pain is being experienced at a conscious level.

Table 2.10. Functions and posture of extremities in vegetative patients

	Percentage of n		
	June 1973 ($n = 110$)	June 1974 ($n = 64$)	June 1976 ($n = 38$)
Quadriplegia	43.1	43.8	55.3
Triplegia	2.8	14.1	5.3
Paraplegia	5.5	9.4	7.9
Hemiplegia	17.4	12.5	18.4
Diplegia	0.9	0	2.6
Monoplegia	0.9	1.6	2.6
Contracture of joints	64.8	79.7	89.5
Spasticity	32.4	21.9	23.7
Rigidity	46.3	50.0	47.4
Decerebrate rigidity	31.2	9.4	10.5

From Higashi et al. (1) with permission.

These patients may also groan and occasionally shout without provocation but no recognizable words are uttered or even mouthed. Some patients smile, frown and occasionally laugh or weep. However, these emotional behaviours show no consistent relation to an appropriate stimulus. Carers frequently report that patients show agitation or other signs of discomfort when the bladder is full or when they have wet themselves or are otherwise uncomfortable. Others claim that patients seem more relaxed when family members arrive and speak or when they stroke them, and become more agitated when they leave; they consider these to be emotional responses indicative of some awareness. However, such behaviours are common in patients who, over a long period of follow-up, show no other signs of awareness or cognition, and most skilled observers accept them as part of the extensive repertoire of reflex responses shown by some vegetative patients. One report described a patient who after 3 years of unresponsiveness began to respond consistently by laughter to the same cartoon film, but 2 years later this remained his only responsive behaviour (17). Higashi found emotional expression in 31% of cases at initial examination and 47% after 3 years, and used this as a basis for classifying some patients as being in a higher grade of vegetative state than others. However, such emotional behaviours showed no correlation with later recovery of consciousness or mortality.

Intermittent episodes of complex behaviour were observed by Schiff et al. in three patients who were vegetative by all other criteria (18,19). Laboratory tests showed that all three had a whole-brain-averaged global metabolism level below 50% of normal. One patient, 20 years vegetative, uttered single words from a vocabulary of four or five once every 48 hours or more; she had preserved islands of less-decreased (but still low) metabolism in the left posterior frontal and temporal lobes. The second, vegetative for 6 months, frequently expressed coordinated but nonpurposeful movements in the arms and/or legs for several hours each day. Metabolism was less decreased (but still low) in the prefrontal and temporal areas. The third, 7 years vegetative, responded to loud noise or attempts at nursing care by clenched teeth, rigid extremities and high-pitched screaming behaviour that abated in response to soothing voices or music. His average cerebral metabolism was only 30% of normal, but it was higher in several right hemisphere regions and he had evoked potentials on magnetometry indicating early and late sensory processing. The conclusion was that these patients had isolated segregated corticothalamic networks that retained connectivity and partial functional integrity. This team has also observed some preserved cortical metabolism in two other patients who had no behaviours outside those of the classical vegetative state (20). One of them had only islands of cortical activity but the other had virtually normal cortical metabolism throughout the brain, but there was severe damage in the thalamus on both sides. Others have recorded laboratory evidence of residual cortical activity in vegetative patients (21). Some patients accepted as vegetative have had repeated episodes of tonic–clonic epilepsy (pp. 161, 162), and this might seem to be evidence of some cortical activity. The conclusion is that consciousness depends on the integrity of sufficient thalamocortical and intercortical connections and that isolated neural activity involving parts of the cortex, even when associated with minimal stereotyped behavioural expression, need not indicate even minimal consciousness (20,22).

Both the ANA and the Task Force definitions refer to brain-stem reflexes being variably intact but the only data from a series are those of Higashi (Tables 2.8 and 2.9). Wide variations in the oculovestibular reflexes have been reported in series of patients and these are reflected in some diagnostic statements. In a series of vegetative patients who died 3–6 weeks after a hypoxic insult six had tonic responses and four unsustained nystagmus (23). In a series of 29 patients who were vegetative from chronic disease four had normal nystagmus, two nystagmus to one side and four had tonic responses (24). The AMA reported that most vegetative patients show tonic responses (10), the Task Force that responses are limited (7), whilst the AAN stated that the reflex is variably preserved (9). Absence of nystagmus was one of the 'other' criteria proposed by the Royal College in London, but this has been challenged as being irrelevant to awareness (p. 162).

Comments about swallowing vary considerably and are of some interest in relation to the debate about whether reliance on tube feeding should be necessary for diagnosis. The Task Force concluded that most patients preserve the swallowing reflex but that coordination is impaired (7), whilst the ANA noted only that swallowing may be preserved (6). Bernat, by contrast, maintained that coordinated medullary and pontine functions are absent in vegetative patients so that swallowing is impossible (25), whilst Tresch et al. (26) accepted only cases with tube feeding into his series. By contrast, Higashi recorded 'swallowing movements' in half of his cases at first examination and in 82% after 3 years; moreover, 26% of his patients were recorded as being fed orally (1). In the review of 847 children in California, identified as probably vegetative by a questionnaire (p. 10), more than a third were said to be fed orally (5). Whether or not vegetative patients are deemed to require tube feeding may be a matter of practicality rather than of pathophysiology. Many who have some capacity to swallow are unable to take in sufficient nourishment for their needs in a reasonable period of time without at least supplemental tube feeding.

It is widely held that vegetative patients are unaware of their surroundings or of themselves, implying loss of the capacity to experience pain or suffering. This was stated unequivocally by the Academy of Neurology in 1989 (9) and was supported by the AMA in 1990 (10), by the ANA in 1993 (6) and by the Task Force in 1994 (7). Three pieces of evidence were considered to support this assertion. One is that observers do not believe that these patients show any behavioural response that indicates pain or suffering. The second is the depression of the cerebral metabolic rate for glucose to levels equivalent to deep surgical anaesthesia in vegetative patients (p. 27). The third is that pathological examination shows such extensive bilateral damage to the cerebral hemispheres or their connections with the thalamus that the structural mechanisms for such experience are no longer available (see Chapter 4).

However, responses to a questionnaire to adult neurologists by the ANA in 1990 indicated that 6% thought that some patients might experience pain, whilst 31% were uncertain; 5% thought that some might experience suffering, whilst 26% were uncertain about this (ANA, unpublished data). A survey of child neurologists (3) revealed that 20% believed that vegetative children could experience pain and suffering, and 75% medicated such children accordingly. Of a group of over 300 neurologists and nursing home directors, 13% believed vegetative patients might have some awareness and 30% that they might experience pain (27). However, a commentator on this study noted the incoherence in many of the responses and suggested that they indicated that the wakeful appearance of these patients was overriding knowledge of their capabilities (28). The Task Force (7) was circumspect about this issue, emphasizing that, whilst the conscious experience of another person can be inferred only by observing their behaviour, there must be a limit to our certainty about this. Those caring for a number of vegetative patients emphasize the importance of exploring all possible avenues of communication before deciding that a patient is showing no signs of cognitive interaction. The theoretical possibility that a patient who is believed to be vegetative might retain some awareness without behavioural evidence of this can never be completely ruled out. An American psychiatrist has robustly criticized the assumption that all vegetative patients are necessarily unconscious or completely unaware, but he does not believe that this diagnosis need exclude patients with only residual, transient, dim awareness (29). An Australian lawyer is similarly critical but is less forgiving about the possibility that pain in these patients may be inadequately treated (30). An American neurologist has reviewed the question of pain from a physiological viewpoint, and argues that an observer cannot know for certain that a vegetative patient cannot perceive pain (31). The relevance of evidence of residual, fragmentary cortical activity to awareness has already been discussed (pp. 11–14, 17). There is great current interest in research into the nature and mechanisms of consciousness, as reflected in there being a *Journal of Consciousness Studies*, and there is an American university centre devoted to such studies that has over 700 papers on its website (32). The question of what vegetative patients actually experience is likely to remain a matter of debate for some time.

The confidence of the diagnosis of the vegetative state

This issue was raised by Bernat, who reported the disagreement between neurologists about the diagnosis in *Nancy Jobes*, who was the subject of a widely reported legal case in the USA (25). She was 29 years old and had been vegetative for 5 years since a cardiac arrest during surgery and had been shown on positron emission tomography (PET) scanning to have only 40% of the normal glucose metabolism in the cerebral cortex. Two of four neurologists experienced in assessing altered conscious states recorded a response to visual threat, two that she made eye contact for a few seconds, one that she had no visual pursuit and one that she had nystagmus. Two neurologists declared that she was not vegetative and the other two that she was. In the event, the judge examined the patient personally and decided to accept that she was vegetative and allowed treatment withdrawal.

In his commentary, Bernat noted the subjective nature of the assessment of whether a patient exhibits evidence of consciousness and noted that responsiveness can vary from time to time according to metabolic or toxic factors, drugs or fatigue. Indeed, those reporting deterioration to the vegetative state in chronic, progressive conditions stress that before becoming permanently vegetative such patients may temporarily go into this state due to infection, heart failure or other systemic illness or from sedative or neuroleptic drugs (24). It was suggested that such patients should be diagnosed as in a persistent vegetative state only when they had been in this state for a month without any complicating factors. There has, however, been a report of a 69-year-old man who became vegetative after cardiac arrest but who, during the remaining 9 months of his life, would become somewhat lucid for some 2 days every 6 weeks (33). These periods, when he would obey a few commands but made no attempt to communicate, were believed to coincide with better control of his systemic and metabolic complications. It was suggested that this phenomenon should be termed a **remitting** vegetative state but this term seems not to have been adopted by anyone else.

A distinctive group of patients that it is important not mistakenly to diagnose as being vegetative are those who are in a de-efferented state, termed the **locked-in syndrome** by Plum and Posner (34). As a result of a lesion in the pons, usually focal ischaemia but very occasionally from trauma to the head or neck (35,36), the descending motor pathways from the brain are out of action. Although sensation and consciousness are fully preserved the patient is paralysed, unable to move or speak; two-thirds can breathe without assistance (35). Limited eye movements are usually possible and the patient can blink so that it is possible for the patient to communicate using a yes/no code based on these residual movements. Skilled neurologists seldom have difficulty in distinguishing this condition from the vegetative state, and, in any event, the history of causation is usually quite different.

The question of mistaken diagnosis of the vegetative state has been explored in three reports. In the first, in four nursing homes in Milwaukee, 62 patients were identified by nurses and physicians as being vegetative but on examination by an expert 11 were considered to show some signs of awareness (26). Two of these 11 were noted to have improved since they had been classified as vegetative on admission to a nursing home, making the error rate 15%. Verified vegetative cases made up only 3% of the 1611 patients in these nursing homes at that time (1991), emphasizing the relative rarity of the condition and that few nursing-home staff can be expected to attain the expertise required for a competent diagnosis.

The second report was of 49 patients referred to a Texas neurorehabilitation unit from acute hospitals, other rehabilitation units and nursing homes with a preadmission diagnosis of coma or persistent vegetative state (37). Over the 7 days following admission to this special unit 18 patients (37%) were considered to show evidence of cognitive responsiveness. Only half of these patients were recognized on transfer as not being vegetative and in more than a fifth it took more than 4 days for the special unit to correct the diagnosis. There were 34 features in these 18 patients that were taken to indicate cognitive responsiveness (Table 2.11) but it was not reported how many patients had only one of these. Patients who showed only 'purposeful' visual responses might have been considered by other observers to have been still vegetative. This and the time taken to recognize responsiveness make this high rate of misdiagnosis somewhat less alarming than it might have seemed at first sight. Misdiagnosis was more common in patients seen more than 3 months since brain insult (41% vs. 29%) and in traumatic than in nontraumatic cases (41% vs. 27%). This report was written before the consensus statements of the ANA (6) and the Task Force (7). Commenting on the ANA report, Celesia (38) noted that until then there had been confusion about terminology and about the medical criteria for diagnosis. He believed that the publication of authoritative statements would clarify the situation and he hoped that any public perception of

Table 2.11. Evidence of cognitive awareness in 18 mistakenly diagnosed as PVS

Obeyed commands	13
Purposeful visual responses	13
Yes/no responses	5
Smiling at jokes	3

From Childs et al. (37).

uncertainty and disagreement about the nosological entity of the persistent vegetative state could be avoided.

The third report came from the Royal Hospital for Neurodisability in London that has a special unit for patients with severe brain damage (39). Its importance lay in the amount of detail provided about the 17 misdiagnosed patients, who accounted for 43% of 40 referred patients said to be in a persistent vegetative state. The age range was 18 to 64 years and ten had sustained traumatic brain damage. Ten had been considered vegetative for 6–12 months, four for 1–2 years and three for 5–7 years. Analysis of 16 cases showed that in only six was responsiveness detected within a week of transfer, in eight it took 8–16 days, in one 40 days and one 175 days. Consistent responses (9/10 times) were recorded in five cases 2–6 weeks after transfer and in six only after 7–25 weeks. Responses were mostly by operating a buzzer (once for yes and twice for no) by movement of a finger, arm or shoulder, or by looking at a named object or letter. Two-thirds of the patients were blind or severely visually impaired, and their inability to show visual fixation or tracking or response to a visual threat was considered possibly to have contributed to their misdiagnosis. The other factor was the very limited motor power available for responses and it often took time even after transfer to recognize that they could respond. None of these patients became able to speak or to dispense with tube feeding. Although some did not become oriented in time and place, several were able to write a letter by responding to a letter board or to a spoken alphabet and to do simple mental arithmetic. In an accompanying commentary Cranford (40) questioned whether, in view of the delay before consistent responses were reported, some cases were not late recoveries rather than late discoveries of consciousness.

Clearly, the diagnosis of the vegetative state should be made only after an adequate period of observation, with due attention to any factors that might temporarily reduce responsiveness. A second expert medical opinion is a wise precaution and indeed is required by some authorities and legal jurisdictions before allowing treatment withdrawal. Such doctors should rely not only on their own observations (necessarily over a limited period) but should seek also information face to face from those who have been caring for the patient over several weeks, including nurses and family (12). The first signs of recovery are often observed by family, nurses or therapists. Claims by them to have noticed meaningful responses must always be investigated carefully with a willingness to revise the diagnosis, although these often prove to have been based on wishful thinking about improvement because of overoptimistic interpretation of reflex activity by those close to the patient.

The minimally conscious state

Some vegetative patients regain consciousness after a time and it is important to recognize such recovery by defining what degree of responsiveness is required for its determination. Initially such patients can be difficult to distinguish from those who are still vegetative and whilst for some this is a transient phase on the way to more substantial recovery others remain like this indefinitely. It was initially suggested that this should be termed the minimally **responsive** state (41) but as all vegetative patients have reflex responses this seems misleading. The preferred term is the minimally **conscious** state, which is more appropriate because the crucial distinction between this and the vegetative state is evidence of cognitive function. Diagnostic criteria for this state have recently been proposed by a group of experts (42). They recognized that it might be considered problematic to designate certain behaviours as markers of consciousness, as these criteria do (Table 2.12), but maintained that there was no better standard against which to judge that a person with such limited responsiveness was conscious. For example, there was still some doubt as to whether visual tracking alone indicates awareness because it has been observed in some patients who remain vegetative by all other criteria for many years (p. 13). The same applied to the patient who repeatedly spoke a few words but was regarded as vegetative by all other criteria over a period of 20 years (p. 17). In eliciting these responses it is important to ensure that the patient is adequately aroused, and that the responses expected are within the motor capacity of the patient but are not of a kind that are already occurring as

Table 2.12. Criteria for the minimally conscious state

Evidence of limited but **clearly discernible** self or environmental awareness on a reproducible or sustained basis, by one or more of these behaviours:

1. Simple command following
2. Gestural or verbal 'yes/no' responses (regardless of accuracy)
3. Intelligible verbalization
4. Purposeful behaviour including movements or affective behaviours in contingent relation to relevant stimuli; examples include:
   (a) appropriate smiling or crying to relevant visual or linguistic stimuli
   (b) response to linguistic content of questions by vocalisation or gesture
   (c) reaching for objects in appropriate direction and location
   (d) touching or holding objects by accommodating to size and shape
   (e) sustained visual fixation or tracking as response to moving stimuli

---

From Giacino et al. (42).

reflex behaviours. It may be necessary to develop communication aids such as a buzzer before responsiveness can be detected.

It is difficult to define when a patient should be regarded as having a higher degree of cognitive functioning than can be termed minimally conscious. The expert group suggested that this might be recognized when there was reliable and consistent functional interactive communication, and/or functional use of more than one object. Communication should include orientation in place and the capacity to give accurate autobiographical information. In one reported case it took two whole day sessions with two psychologists on two occasions to establish that a patient with very limited responsiveness was able to give quite detailed autobiographical data and to learn some simple tasks (43,44). In a commentary on this case a rehabilitationist referred to her as being minimally conscious (45) and this led to considerable controversy about whether this was a correct designation (J. Giacino, personal communication). Some maintained that her cognitive function made her better than this, whilst others considered that if it took so much expert effort to establish her capabilities it could hardly be called functional interactive communication in a practical sense.

Laboratory investigations

Electroencephalogram (EEG)

A wide range of abnormalities have been found which makes this an unhelpful investigation either for the diagnosis of, or the prognosis for recovery from, the vegetative state. A number of studies dealt not with diagnosis, but with attempts to predict which patients would become vegetative by using the findings in the early stages after acute brain insults. However, these attempts were unsuccessful. There have been only a few studies that reported findings in substantial series of vegetative patients (1,23,46,47). The commonest abnormalities were delta or theta rhythms that were usually unreactive to stimuli, were often paroxysmal and were sometimes asymmetrical. Between 10% and 20% of cases have shown near-normal alpha rhythm late in their course, but again this was often unreactive to sensory stimuli. Some cases had very low amplitude records and about 5% an isoelectric record, which had sometimes persisted for over 2 years. Neither the transition from coma to the vegetative state, nor recovery of consciousness after being vegetative, have been accompanied by consistent changes in the EEG. Indeed, Higashi et al. (1) found several cases in whom the EEG improved without clinical change and others in whom clinical improvement was associated with an unchanged or even a deteriorated EEG.

The brain-stem auditory-evoked response was usually normal but the somatosensory-evoked response was often absent or shows prolonged central conduction time. However, normal responses were recorded in some patients who remained vegetative, whilst some degree of cognitive activity can occur in some patients with absent responses. It is presumed that, like the variability of reflex clinical responses, these findings reflect the patchy anatomical distribution of the brain damage, which has, however, been enough in aggregate to produce the vegetative state.

Neuroimaging

Computerized tomography (CT) scanning or magnetic resonance imaging (MRI) of the brain of the vegetative patient shows severe brain atrophy with enlarged ventricles and, when the lesion is cortical, enlargement also of the subarachnoid spaces over the cortex. However, similar degrees of atrophy have been found in age-matched patients with severe dementia who have some cognitive function (24). Late imaging may also show atrophy of the thalamus, but this was also a pathological feature of some head injured patients who were conscious with severe disability (p. 52). There is therefore no radiological appearance that is diagnostic for the vegetative state. However, lack of progressive or marked atrophy may indicate potential for recovery, and this was a feature of two frequently quoted cases of late recovery (48,49). Some developmental abnormalities in children produce characteristic radiological pictures, but again no particular degree of abnormality can be equated with the vegetative state, although it may indicate lack of potential for recovery.

In a series of patients who were vegetative 6 weeks after head injury an attempt was made to correlate the MRI findings at that time with whether or not the patients had recovered consciousness after 1 year (50,51). Although more of the patients who remained vegetative had radiological evidence of severe diffuse axonal injury this was a feature of a quarter of the patients who recovered to some degree, thus confirming our finding of considerable overlap in the neuropathological features in the brains of vegetative and severely disabled patients (p. 52).

Developments in functional MRI make it possible to measure the level of activity in certain parts of the brain and to correlate these findings with evidence of cognitive function. This is still at the level of research rather than routine clinical diagnosis.

Cerebral blood flow (CBF)

A number of studies have shown reduced CBF in vegetative patients. This applied to all four patients in an early study using the Xenon technique (52), and to all seven patients in a PET study (53). Using another method, local reduction of CBF (most marked frontally) was found in the first 4 months in four out of six vegetative patients who showed no recovery after 1–5 years, but in none of the six who did recover (54). In one patient who was vegetative following hypoglycaemic brain damage an abnormally high flow was found at 6 and 34 months (55). In view of this case and the two in the previous study who remained vegetative with a normal CBF it is clear that CBF alone is of limited diagnostic value, although a very low flow provides supportive evidence of the vegetative state.

Positron emission tomography (PET)

Several studies of cerebral glucose oxidative metabolism using this technique in vegetative patients (17) have shown average levels between 35% of normal (postanoxic) and 56% (post-traumatic). These average values are lower than in experimental and clinical studies of deep anaesthesia (53). One study compared seven vegetative patients with three in the locked-in syndrome and 18 normal volunteers (53). The vegetative patients (one traumatic and six anoxic) were 3 weeks to 68 months since insult, the locked-in patients 14 weeks to 15 months. The metabolic activity was 40% of normal in the vegetative patients and 75% in those locked-in, with no overlap between the two groups. This reduction in activity was found not only in the cerebral cortex but also in the basal ganglia and cerebellum. This marked reduction compares with only 13% reduction during nondreaming sleep in normal volunteers. Another study examined seven vegetative patients, five severely disabled but conscious patients and 16 normal volunteers (56). All patients had suffered anoxic brain damage at least one month previously, with four already showing cortical atrophy on CT scan. The mean reduction in metabolism was 54% in the vegetative patients and 38% in the severely disabled. However, two of the severely disabled patients had lower metabolic rates than the highest of the vegetative patients, but the low rates in these two conscious patients were associated with very poor recoveries.

In the patients of Plum et al. (18) who were vegetative but had some fragments of complex behaviour the average levels were very low but there were some areas that had slightly higher (but still very low) levels of cortical metabolism. In the study of Tommasino et al. (57) some areas of the brain in vegetative patients had 71% of normal metabolism. The more extended studies of Schiff et al. have found virtually normal metabolism in most of the cortex in one patient whose damage was localized to the thalamus and who had been vegetative for 6 years (20). From these studies it seems that even PET may not be a completely reliable test, although low values are strongly supportive. It has been suggested that the response of the metabolic rate to external stimuli might make it more discriminative (21,25). However, the restricted availability of this technology to a few research institutions limits its value as a practical diagnostic tool.

None of the recent statements on the diagnosis of the vegetative state require any radiological or laboratory investigations. Some specify that these are of little help in confirming the diagnosis. This is because, with the exception of the very low metabolic activity found in most vegetative cases with PET scanning, none of these tests directly reflects consciousness

What duration for definition?

The original description did not indicate how soon a vegetative state might be termed persistent, and it was careful to state that no data were yet available on the interval after which the condition might be deemed permanent (8). The data now available on prognosis for recovery are discussed in Chapter 5. Neurosurgeons who have reported on patients deemed vegetative 1 month after injury (58,59,60) have emphasized that substantial numbers of these regain consciousness and that some recover well. Neurologists have analysed the outcome of patients diagnosed vegetative at 1 day and 7 days after a nontraumatic insult (13,61). Some epidemiological reports have been limited to patients who have been in this state for 3 or 6 months (see Chapter 3). The ANA Report (6) proposed that persistent vegetative state be applied only to patients who had been **in this state** for 1 month. The Task Force (7), however, accepted those who were vegetative at 1 month **after an acute insult**. Those in whom the causation was a chronic brain condition had to have been vegetative for 1 month to be classified as in a persistent vegetative state. As most traumatic cases do not open their eyes for 2–3 weeks after injury the ANA definition would exclude some of the surgical cases diagnosed one month after injury but who had recovered after less than a month in a vegetative state. Prognosis based on the diagnosis of a vegetative state at **1 month after injury** will therefore be more optimistic than in cases that have been in a vegetative state **for 1 month**, but this difference will be of little significance after 3–6 months. However, the occasional statement that persistent vegetative state cannot be diagnosed until a patient has been vegetative for a year betrays confusion between diagnosis and prognosis.

REFERENCES

1 Higashi K, Sakata Y, Hatano M et al. Epidemiological studies on patients with a persistent vegetative state. *J Neurol Neurosurg Psychiatry* 1977; 40: 870–78

2 Sato S, Imamura H, Ueki K et al. Epidemiological survey of vegetative state patients

in the Tokohu District, Japan. *Neurol Med Chir (Tokyo)* 1978; 18: 141–5

3 Ashwal S, Bale JF, Coulter DL et al. The persistent vegetative state in children. Report of the Child Neurology Society Ethics Committee. *Ann Neurol* 1992; 32: 570–76

4 Nelson WA, Bernat JL. Decisions to withhold or terminate treatment. In: Bernat JL, ed. *Neurological Clinics. Ethical Issues in Neurologic Practice. Vol 7*. Philadelphia: WB Saunders 1989: 759–74

5 Ashwal S, Eyman RK, Call TL. Life expectancy of children in a persistent vegetative state. *Pediatric Neurol* 1994; 10: 27–33

6 American Neurological Association Committee on Ethical Affairs. Persistent vegetative state. *Ann Neurol* 1993; 33: 386–90

7 The Multi-Society Task Force on the Persistent Vegetative State. Statement on medical aspects of the persistent vegetative state. *N Engl J Med* 1994; 330: 1499–508

8 Jennett B, Plum F. Persistent vegetative state after brain damage. A syndrome in search of a name. *Lancet* 1972; 1: 734–7

9 American Academy of Neurology. Position of the American Academy of Neurology on certain aspects of the care and management of the persistent vegetative state patient. *Neurology* 1989; 39: 125–6

10 American Medical Association Council on Scientific Affairs and Council on Ethical and Judicial Affairs. Persistent vegetative state and the decision to withdraw or withhold life support. *JAMA* 1990; 263: 426–30

11 Quality Standards Subcommittee of the American Academy of Neurology. Practice parameters: Assessment and management of patients in the persistent vegetative state. *Neurology* 1995; 45: 1015–18

12 Royal College of Physicians Working Group. The permanent vegetative state. *J R Coll Physicians Lond* 1996; 30: 119–21

13 Levy DE, Bates D, Caronna JJ et al. Prognosis in nontraumatic coma. *Ann Intern Med* 1981; 94: 293–301

14 Plum F, Posner JB. *The Diagnosis of Stupor and Coma* 3rd Edn. Philadelphia: FA Davis, 1980

15 Giacino JT, Kalmar K. The vegetative and minimally conscious states: a comparison of clinical features and functional outcome. *J Head Trauma Rehabil* 1997; 12: 36–51

16 Andrews K. International Working Party on the Management of the Vegetative State: summary report. *Brain Injury* 1996; 10: 797–806

17 Andrews K. Recovery of patients after four months or more in a persistent vegetative state. *BMJ* 1993; 306: 1597–9

18 Plum F, Schiff N, Ribary U et al. Coordinated expression in chronically unconscious patients. *Philos Trans R Soc Lond B Biol Sci* 1998; 353: 1929–33

19 Schiff N, Ribary U, Plum F et al. Words without mind. *J Cogn Neurosci* 1999; 11: 650–56

20 Schiff N, Ribary U, Moreno D et al. Residual cerebral activity and behavioral

fragments can remain in the persistently vegetative state, *Brain.* In press

21 Menon DK, Owen AM, Williams EJ et al. Cortical processing in persistent vegetative state. *Lancet* 1999; 352: 200

22 Schiff N, Plum F. Cortical function in the persistent vegetative state. *Trends Cogn Sci* 1999; 3: 43–6

23 Dougherty JH, Rawlinson DG, Levy DE et al. Hypoxic-ischemic brain injury and the vegetative state: Clinical and neuropathologic correlation. *Neurology* 1981; 31: 991–7

24 Walshe TM, Leonard C. Persistent vegetative state. Extension of the syndrome to include chronic disorders. *Arch Neurol* 1985; 42: 1045–7

25 Bernat JL. The boundaries of the persistent vegetative state. *J Clin Ethics* 1992; 3: 176–80

26 Tresch DD, Sims FH, Duthie EH et al. Clinical characteristics of patients in the persistent vegetative state. *Arch Intern Med* 1991; 151: 930–32

27 Payne K, Taylor RM, Stocking C et al. Physicians' attitudes about the care of patients in the persistent vegetative state. *Ann Intern Med* 1996; 125: 104–10

28 Cassell EJ. Clinical incoherence about persons: the problem of the persistent vegetative state. *Ann Intern Med* 1996; 125: 146–7

29 Howsepian AA. The 1994 Multi-Society Task Force consensus statement on the persistent vegetative state; a critical analysis. *Issues Law Med* 1996; 12: 3–29

30 Borthwick CJ. The permanent vegetative state; ethical crux, medical fiction? *Issues Law Med* 1996; 12: 167–85

31 McQuillen MP. Can people who are unconscious or in the 'vegetative state' perceive pain? *Issues Law Med* 1991; 6: 373–83

32 Tonks A. Persistent vegetative state (Website of the week) *BMJ* 2001; 322: 371

33 Thomasma DC, Brumlik J. Ethical issues in the treatment of patients with a remitting vegetative state. *Am J Med* 1984; 77: 373–7

34 Plum F, Posner JB. *Diagnosis of stupor and coma.* Philadelphia: FA Davis, 1966

35 Patterson JR, Grabois M. Locked-in syndrome: A review of 139 cases. *Stroke* 1986; 17: 758–64

36 Keane JR. Locked-in syndrome after head and neck trauma. *Neurology* 1986; 36: 80–82

37 Childs NL, Mercer WN, Childs HW. Accuracy of diagnosis of persistent vegetative state. *Neurology* 1993; 43: 1465–7

38 Celesia GG. Persistent vegetative state. *Neurology* 1993; 43: 1457–8

39 Andrews K, Murphy L, Munday R et al. Misdiagnosis of the vegetative state: retrospective study in a rehabilitation unit. *BMJ* 1996; 313: 13–16

40 Cranford R. Misdiagnosis of the persistent vegetative state: An apparently high rate of misdiagnosis demands critical review and action. *BMJ* 1996; 313: 5–6

41 American Congress of Rehabilitation Medicine. Recommendations for use of uniform nomenclature pertinent to patients with severe alterations of consciousness.

Arch Phys Med Rehabil 1995; 76: 205–9

42 Giacino J, Ashwal S, Childs N et al. The minimally conscious state: definition and diagnostic criteria. *Neurology* 2001; 57: in press

43 McMillan TM. Neuropsychological assessment after extremely severe head injury in a case of life or death. *Brain Injury* 1997; 11: 483–90

44 Shiel A, Wilson BA. Assessment of extremely severe head injury in a case of life or death: further support for McMillan. *Brain Injury* 1998; 12: 809–16

45 Phipps E, Whyte J. Medical decision-making with persons who are minimally conscious. *Am J Phys Med Rehabil* 1999; 78: 77–82

46 Hansotia PL. Persistent vegetative state: review and report of electrodiagnostic studies in eight cases. *Arch Neurol* 1985; 42: 1048–52

47 Danze F, Brule JF, Haddad K. Chronic vegetative state after severe head injury. *Neurosurg Rev* 1989; 12: 477–99

48 Rosenberg GA, Johnson SF, Brenner RP. Recovery of cognition after prolonged vegetative state. *Ann Neurol* 1977; 2: 167–8

49 Snyder BD, Cranford RE, Rubens AB et al. Delayed recovery from post-anoxic persistent vegetative state. *Ann Neurol* 1983; 14: 152

50 Kampfl A, Schumutzhard E, Franz G et al. Prediction of recovery from posttraumatic vegetative state with cerebral magnetic resonance imaging. *Lancet* 1998; 351: 1763–7

51 Kampfl A, Franz G, Aichner F et al. PVS after closed head injury: MRI in 42 patients. *J Neurosurg* 1998; 88: 809–16

52 Ingvar DH. Cerebral blood flow and metabolism in complete apallic syndromes, in states of severe dementia and in akinetic mutism. *Acta Neurol Scand* 1973; 49: 233–44

53 Levy DE, Sidtis JJ, Rottenberg DA et al. Differences in cerebral blood flow and glucose utilization in vegetative versus locked-in patients. *Ann Neurol* 1987; 22: 673–82

54 Oder W, Goldenberg C, Podreka I et al. HM-PAO-SPECT in persistent vegetative state after head injury: prognostic indicator of the likelihood of recovery? *Intensive Care Med* 1991; 17: 149–53

55 Agardh CD, Rosen I, Ryding E. Persistent vegetative state with high cerebral blood flow following profound hypoglycaemia. *Ann Neurol* 1983; 14: 482–6

56 DeVolder AG, Goffinet AM, Bol A et al. Brain glucose metabolism in postanoxic syndrome. Positron emission tomographic study. *Arch Neurol* 1990; 47: 197–204

57 Tommasino C, Grana C, Lucignani G et al. Regional cerebral metabolism in comatose and vegetative state patients *J Neurosurg Anesthesiol* 1995; 7: 109–16

58 Braakman R, Jennett B, Minderhoud JM. Prognosis of the posttraumatic vegetative state. *Acta Neurochir (Wein)* 1988; 95: 49–52

59 Levin HS, Saydjari C, Eisenberg HM et al. Vegetative state after closed head injury. A traumatic Coma Data Bank Report. *Arch Neurol* 1991; 580–85

60 Sazbon L, Groswasser Z. Outcome in 134 patients with prolonged posttraumatic unawareness. *J Neurosurg* 1990; 72: 75–80

61 Levy DE, Knill-Jones RP, Plum F. The vegetative state and its prognosis following non-traumatic coma. *Ann NY Acad Sci* 1978; 315: 293–306

3

Epidemiology

Frequency

No routinely-collected statistics provide data about patients in PVS because this syndrome is not recognized by the International Classification of Diseases. Information comes either from clinical series of patients in acute care facilities with traumatic or nontraumatic coma, some of whom become vegetative, and of patients with an established vegetative state in long-term care, or from planned surveys of vegetative patients in various institutions in a defined community. Estimates of the frequency of vegetative cases and of the distribution of causes vary widely according to the source of the data, and not all distinguish clearly between incidence (new cases per year) and prevalence (cases extant at any one time). A major problem is that vegetative patients are distributed in many different types of institution including acute hospitals, geriatric or young chronic sick units, mental hospitals, rehabilitation units, nursing homes and charitable care facilities. A significant number of vegetative patients are cared for at home. Of 847 vegetative children in a Californian study (1), 25% were being cared for at home, as were about half of 458 cases identified in the UK by responses to a telephone helpline following a television programme on the vegetative state in 1994. Patients at home will not be discovered by surveys of institutions.

Differences of definition are another source of variation in estimates of frequency (Tables 2.1–2.6). How long patients had to have been vegetative for inclusion in a survey has varied from 2 weeks (2) to 6 months (3). One month after head injury vegetative survivors are three to four times more common than after 6 months, because by 6 months many of those who were vegetative at 1 month have either died or are no longer vegetative. It is therefore not surprising that both incidence and prevalence rates range widely in different reports.

Surveys of prevalence

Higashi et al. sent enquiries to 269 hospitals in Japan in 1973 and received notification of 193 possible cases from 189 hospitals (4). When patients were then examined by the investigators only 110 (57%) proved to meet the criteria – a warning that ascertainment by mail order is inherently unreliable. This study ranged over 16 prefectures but there were 37 cases from the one prefecture where all hospitals responded and this was the basis of the estimate of 25 per million population (PMP) for the prevalence of patients vegetative for at least 3 months. All diagnoses were included, with some developmental and degenerative conditions.

Sato et al. (5) also required 3 months in the vegetative state and sent questionnaires to 759 hospitals in seven prefectures in 1975; the response rate averaged 78% but the estimate of 25 PMP was based on prefectures from which all hospitals responded. As the motivation for this enquiry was to identify patients receiving financial aid from local authorities, it was limited to patients who had previously been 'leading a useful life' – in effect this meant only patients who had suffered acute brain insults, and a very small proportion of children (6%). The authors referred to two other surveys, published in Japanese only, which had yielded rates of 23 PMP, very similar to their own and that of Higashi. A repeat survey in one of these regions in 1997 found that the prevalence had increased to 44 PMP (6).

Minderhoud and Braakman (3) sent questionnaires to 480 Dutch hospitals and nursing homes in 1983 and received an 80% response. The 53 patients identified as vegetative for at least 6 months after an acute brain insult led them to estimate at least 5 PMP in the Netherlands. By extrapolation this would mean 7.6 PMP at 3 months (p. 38), much lower than the Japanese figure. An alternative basis for estimating the prevalence of vegetative patients from acute causes in the Netherlands was a report from the Royal Dutch Medical Association on withdrawal of treatment from patients in 'prolonged coma' (7). This was recommended after 3–6 months for traumatic cases and 1 month for nontraumatic and it was estimated that such decisions would be required for 100 cases a year in the whole country. This would represent a prevalence of 6.7 PMP.

A study of 18 regions in France in 1987 yielded 483 patients who had been vegetative for at least 3 months, giving a rate of 14 PMP (8). However, the regional rate ranged from 5 to 33 PMP. Elsewhere in the book that reported this study there is also an estimate of about 1000 vegetative cases in France as a whole, a rate of 18 PMP.

A survey of the 1600 residents of four nursing homes in Milwaukee, Wisconsin, in 1990 yielded 51 patients verified as vegetative when examined by one of the investigators, which is 3% of the residents (9). Only patients being tube fed were accepted and all were adults who had been vegetative for at least a year. A 1986 US Government Department of Health and Human Services (DHHS) Report quoted by Spudis (10) indicated that there were then 1.4 million beds in the country in nursing homes that provided skilled or intermediate care. Assuming that 1% of patients in these beds were vegetative this would mean 56 vegetative patients PMP. The source of this much lower estimate of the number of vegetative patients in the nursing home population than Tresch had found was not declared.

The Child Neurology Society in the US sent questionnaires in 1991 to 960 members, of whom 250 (26%) responded (11). As well as canvassing opinions about diagnosis and management, respondents were asked to estimate the number of vegetative children seen in a year in a number of diagnostic categories and age ranges. Some 1600 cases who had been vegetative for 3–6 months were reported. If grossed up for all the child neurologists in the US this made 6000 for the country as a whole, a rate of 24 children in a vegetative state PMP. An alternative approach to estimating the prevalence of vegetative survival in children was made in California between 1980 and 1991 (1). This reviewed a register of over 155 000 developmentally disabled California State residents, using items from a standard Client Development Evaluation Report form to identify those judged to be in a vegetative state (Table 2.4). On this basis, 847 patients were deemed to be vegetative (p. 7) and, using the same criteria, their status was confirmed 2 years later. This gave a rate of 29 PMP, not dissimilar from the 24 found by the child neurologists. It is doubtful whether all vegetative patients in a community would be known to a child neurologist or would be on a state disabled register. For these reasons these estimates of prevalence may be on the low side.

In 1990, the AMA made an estimate for the US of 60–100 PMP by applying a modification of the Japanese rates, which were increased (by an undeclared factor) to allow for the wider application in the US of critical care medicine, resuscitation, parenteral feeding and infection control, and to include cases resulting from advanced dementia (12). However, this

Table 3.1. Estimates of prevalence of PVS in US (includes chronic causes)

	Year	Location	PMP
AMA (12)	1990	USA	60–100 (? adults)
Tresch et al. (9)	1991	USA	168 adults
Spudis (10)	1991	USA	56 adults
Ashwal et al. (11)	1992	USA	16–40 children, 40–100 adults, 56–140 all
Ashwal et al. (1)	1994	USA	24–40 children, 40–100 adults, 64–140 all

estimate was made before any of the US surveys described above and no mention was made of children, and this figure was subsequently referred to by the Task Force as applying to adults. In fact the Task Force (13) accepted the estimate of 56–140 PMP of Ashwal et al. (11) that includes children. The wide range in these estimates (Table 3.1) emphasizes the uncertainty that remains about the size of the problem.

Incidence studies

These depend on the follow-up of patients who have suffered acute brain insults, traumatic and nontraumatic. Most studies have been on severe head injuries, which have been a focus of interest in several countries in recent years and for which the Glasgow Outcome Scale is routinely used, thereby identifying vegetative survivors. In these studies a head injury was classified as severe if in coma for more than 6 hours or had a postresuscitation Glasgow Coma Score of 8 or less. Such studies show that 6–16% of such severe injuries are vegetative one month after injury (Table 3.2). During the first year some vegetative patients die and others regain consciousness, so that of those vegetative at one month a decreasing percentage are alive and vegetative at 3, 6 and 12 months (Table 3.3). As a result the proportion of severe head injury admissions who are vegetative falls steadily during the first year (Table 3.4). Some studies have produced data only for patients vegetative at 3 or 6 months but it is possible to extrapolate from these to 1 month or from 1 month to later periods, using the proportions in Table 3.3.

There are few systematic data about the frequency of the vegetative state

Table 3.2. Proportion of severe head injury admissions who are in VS at 1 month

	International study (14) 1970–77				4 UK Centres (15) 1968–88	US Trauma Coma Data Bank (16) 1984–87	France (8) 1991	EBIC (18) 1995
	Glasgow	Netherlands	Los Angeles	Total				
n	788	418	225	1371	114	746 adults		481 adults
Percentage VS at 1 month	7	12	16	10	6.4	14[a]	8–10[b]	16[c]

[a] On discharge from neurosurgery – 46% within 30 days of injury, 79% within 60 days.
[b] Estimate based on 2.5% in vegetative state at 6 months.
[c] Estimate based on 4% at 6 months.

Table 3.3. Proportion of patients in vegetative state at one month who are still vegetative at intervals during the first year (%)

	Braakman (14) HI	Murray (15) HI	Sazbon (17) HI	Task Force (13) HI	Task Force (13) All
n at 1 month	140	68	134	540	754
3 months	35	35	51	56	59
6 months	21	25	32	32	37
12 months	11	–	14	18	24

HI, head injury

Table 3.4. Vegetative survivors at various intervals after severe head injury (%)

Interval	International Study 1968–80 (14) ($n = 1371$)	4 UK Centres 1986–88 (15) ($n = 1114$)
1 month	10	6.4
3 months	3.6	2
6 months	2.2	1.5
12 months	1	–

(VS) after nontraumatic coma, perhaps because the causes are various and the concern of several different specialists. The only sizeable series is that from an Anglo-American collaborative study (19) that comprised 500 adults of whom 12% were vegetative at 1 month (31% of the survivors). Many more of the hypoxic patients became vegetative than patients in coma from other nontraumatic causes (Table 3.5). Of 168 children with nontraumatic coma in London only 3% became vegetative (20). There are no data on the population-based incidence of nontraumatic coma from which an estimate could be made of the incidence of vegetative patients from these causes in the population.

There are now good epidemiological data for the frequency of occurrence and of severity of head injuries in the UK, USA and France (21,22,8), and from these data the annual incidence PMP of vegetative survivors from trauma can be calculated (Tables 3.6, 3.7 and 3.8). For Israel this has been estimated directly at 4 PMP (23). By using data on the proportion of vegetative patients that have resulted from traumatic and nontraumatic insults it is possible to estimate the incidence of vegetative survivors from all acute insults in the UK, USA and France (Tables 3.6, 3.7 and 3.8). The incidence of vegetative survival from all acute causes at 1, 3 and 6 months in the three countries can then be compared (Table 3.9). The higher rates in the US and France reflect the greater frequency of severe head injuries there than in the UK.

Age distribution of vegetative patients

As noted in discussing prevalence rates, the definition of a child is not consistent between reports and in some it is not even clearly stated. The

Table 3.5(a). Vegetative outcome one month after nontraumatic coma

	of all cases		of survivors	
	n	% veg	*n*	% veg
Hypoxia	210	20	92	46
Subarachnoid haemorrhage	38	5	10	20
Other stroke	143	5	37	19
Hepatic	51	2	26	4
Other	58	14	32	25
Total	500	12	195	31

Table 3.5(b). Causes in nontraumatic vegetative cases

	n	%
Hypoxia	42	70
Cerebrovascular	9	15
Hepatic	1	2
Other	8	13
Total	60	

Data from Levy et al. (19).

Table 3.6. Estimated incidence of acute VS in UK
(PMP, per million population)

90 severe HI PMP, 6% VS at 1 month = 5 PMP
if HI = 40% of all acute VS (refs 3,4)
Total VS PMP per year at 1 month = 14
                                3 months = 8 (using Task Force decrement)
                                6 months = 5

Based on data in Jennett (21,22).

upper limit seems to vary between 16, 18 or 20 years. The proportion of 'children' in different series varies from 6% to 38% (Table 3.10). The age distribution within childhood varied between the two American surveys of children (Table 3.11). In the two adult series that included nonacute causes, the age range was 54 to 85 years in the one that excluded injury and

Table 3.7. Estimated incidence of acute VS in USA
(PMP, per million population)

HI death rate = UK × 2.8, assume severe HI admissions also × 2.8
Vegetative rate 14% = UK rate × 2.3
so one month VS rate = 5 × 2.8 × 2.3 = 32.2 PMP from head injury
HI = 70% of acute VS (ref 13)
Total VS PMP per year at 1 month = 46
                              3 months = 27 (using Task Force decrement)
                              6 months = 17

Based on data from Jennett (21,22).

Table 3.8. Estimated incidence of acute VS in France
(PMP, per million population)

---

200 severe HI PMP, 2.5% VS at 6 months = 5 PMP
This = 20 PMP from HI at 1 month (using UK decrement)
HI = 30% of acute VS
Total VS PMP per year at 1 month = 67
                              3 months = 40 (using Task Force decrement)
                              6 months = 25

Based on data from Tasseau et al. (8).

Table 3.9. Estimated incidence PMP from all acute causes

	1 month	3 months	6 months
UK	14	8	5
USA	46	27	17
France	67	40	25

anoxia (24) and in the other was 19 to 96 years (9). In the former, the mean age was 66 years, in the latter, it varied from 85 years for dementia to 28 years for trauma cases. In Higashi's series in 1977, only 26% were over 60 years of age (4), but in a survey of 653 Japanese cases 20 years later, 75% were over 60 and 33% over 80 years of age (6).

Table 3.10. Proportion of children

Cause	%	n	Author	Reference
All	26	110	Higashi	4
All	6	219	Sato	5
Head injury	38	140	Braakman	14
Head injury	26	134	Sazbon	23
Traumatic	20	540	Task Force (cases)	13
Acute nontraumatic	21	214	Task Force (cases)	13
All	29	–	Task Force (estimate)	13
All	29–38	–	Ashwal (estimate)	1

Most studies define children as <18 or 20 years – but Braakman and Sazbon used <15 years.

Table 3.11. Ages in children's surveys

California disabled (1) ($n=847$)		Child neurologists (11) ($n=1491$)	
Age	%	Age	%
<1 year	23	<2 mths	20
1–2 years	13	2 mths–2 years	29
2–6 years	23	2–7 years	30
7–18 years	24	>7 years	21
19+ years	18		

Causes

Acute damage

Only acute brain damage (trauma and ischaemia) was referred to in the original description of PVS. Most reports in the next few years focused on vegetative survival as an outcome of either traumatic or nontraumatic coma, whilst some surveys were also limited to such acute cases.

Table 3.12. Causes in 53 cases vegetative at least 6 months

	%	Mean age (years)
Head injury	45	31.2
Cerebrovascular	40	73.4
Anoxia/hypoglycaemia	15	20.3

Minderhoud and Braakman (3).

Table 3.13. Causes in 110 cases vegetative at least 3 months

	n	% of total	% of acute
Head injury	38	34	41
Cerebrovascular	21	19	23
Cerebral anoxia	12	11	13
Brain tumour	10	9	11
Infection	7	6	8
Intoxication	4	4	4
Total acute	92		
Developmental	14	13	
Degenerative	4	4	
Total	110		

Higashi et al. (4).

Table 3.14. Causes in nursing home series

	n	%	Mean age (years)
Cerebrovascular	17	33	71.9
Dementia	13	25	85.2
Anoxia	10	20	47.9
Cerebral trauma	7	14	28.3
Other	4	8	60.5
Total	51		

Tresch et al. (9).

In the Netherlands acute survey (3) and the acute cases in Higashi's Japanese survey (4), head injury comprised 45% and 41% respectively (Tables 3.12 and 3.13). However, Sato (5) found only 24% due to head injury, explaining this by the decreasing incidence of head injury and the increasing use of active treatment (including surgery) for cerebrovascular accidents. Only 30% of 157 cases in France were attributed to trauma (8). However, in the aggregate series of 754 vegetative cases from acute insults assembled from the literature by the Task Force (13) head injuries accounted for 72% of 603 adults and 70% of 151 children. This high proportion of trauma cases, however, probably reflects the large number of reports of outcome after severe head injury by neurosurgeons during the previous decade or so.

In the only survey of nursing home patients (9), both acute and chronic cases were included and head injury accounted for 14%, anoxia for 20% and cerebrovascular disease for 33% (Table 3.14). This balance between anoxia and cerebrovascular cases was approximately mirrored in the Netherlands and Japanese surveys, but the Anglo-American nontraumatic adult series had many more hypoxic than cerebrovascular cases (Table 3.5).

No reports on vegetative patients describe the different causes of cerebral anoxia that have led to this state. These include cardiac arrest from primary cardiac disease, from medical accidents (mostly under anaesthesia), from respiratory obstruction and episodes of severe hypotension, near drowning or strangulation and carbon monoxide poisoning. Of the 210 cases of hypoxia in the nontraumatic coma series 71% had had cardiac arrest, 18% profound hypotension and 11% respiratory obstruction (19). Among other nontraumatic insults leading to vegetative survival are intracranial infections and tumours, and in diabetics hypoglycaemia with delayed discovery and treatment.

Nonacute conditions

The first reference to the vegetative state after nonacute causes of brain damage was in Higashi's survey of 110 cases in Japan published in 1977 (Table 3.13). This included four cases of degenerative disease and 14 of developmental conditions (amounting to 17% of the cases). No details were given of these cases, nor was comment made that they represented an extension of the aetiological base of this condition beyond acute insults. That, however, was the title of a report from Walshe and Leonard in 1985

Table 3.15. Causes in nonacute series

Alzheimer's	18	51%
Pick's	1	
Huntingdon's	5	14%
Stroke	4	11%
Creutzfeldt–Jakob's	2	
Parkinson's	2	
Degeneration	3	
Demyelinating	1	
Hydrocephalus	1	
Total	37	

Walshe and Leonard (24).

(24), which described 37 cases institutionalized in a Veterans Administration Neurology Service in Massachusetts and excluded those following head injury or anoxia. There was a wide range of causes (Table 3.15), half being cases of Alzheimer's disease. They noted that some patients with advanced dementia who remained ambulant showed no more evidence of higher mental responsiveness than vegetative patients, but considered that these should not be classified as vegetative – a decision underlined as wise in subsequent journal correspondence. In the nursing home series of Tresch (9), 25% of the vegetative patients were in the late stages of a dementing illness (Table 3.14). A more recent review of a small number of patients with Alzheimer's disease suggested, however, that few progress to the vegetative state (25).

Children

A review of 17 vegetative children in 1980 excluded neonates and cases of head trauma (26). Anoxia accounted for 12 and meningitis for another four cases. A British editorial in 1984 noted that paediatricians were beginning to see vegetative patients more often because of the increasing frequency of survival from head injury and cardiac arrest, but that cases also resulted from metabolic and encephalitic coma (27). Systematic data on children has become available from the American Child Neurologists' Survey (11) and that of the California Disabled (1). These two reports use

Table 3.16. Causes in two children's surveys (%)

Child neurologists (11) ($n=1491$)		California disabled (1) ($n=847$)	
Trauma	27	Trauma	15
Infection	23	Infection	10
Asphyxia	23	Nontraumatic	16
Near drowning	13	Perinatal	18
SIDS	2		
Malformations	3	Chromo/develop	13
Other	9	Other	28

SIDS, sudden infant death syndrome.

Table 3.17. Risk of developing PVS from acute severe brain injury in children

Disease	Risk of developing PVS %
Severe traumatic brain injury	5–10
Cardiorespiratory arrest	
In hospital	15
Out of hospital	60–70
Near drowning	20–45
Central nervous system infections	5–10
Haemorrhagic shock encephalopathy	80
Strangulation	50
Sudden infant death syndrome	40

From Ashwal (28) with permission.

different diagnostic categories, which makes comparisons difficult (Table 3.16). In the Child Neurologists' series, 38% were ascribed to causes producing anoxia, while such cases were presumably hidden within the nontraumatic and perinatal categories of the California series. Trauma accounted for 27% of one series and 15% of the other, but the Child Neurologists found that it accounted for 40% of those over 7 years of age. Infection was a much commoner cause than in adults. Malformations accounted for rather few cases in these two surveys. Of 29 cases less than 20 years of age in Higashi's survey, 41% were developmental, 28% anoxic and 21% traumatic (4).

Table 3.18. Aetiologies of PVS in children

Acute insults

Traumatic
1. Nonaccidental injury (i.e. child abuse)
2. Motor vehicle accidents
3. Birth injury
4. Gunshot wounds and other forms of direct cerebral injury

Nontraumatic
1. Hypoxic-ischaemic encephalopathy
   a. Cardiorespiratory arrest
   b. Perinatal asphyxia
   c. Near-drowning
   d. Suffocating/strangulation
2. Cerebrovascular
   a. Cerebral haemorrhage
   b. Cerebral infarction
3. Central nervous system infection
   a. Bacterial meningitis
   b. Viral meningoencephalitis
   c. Brain abscess
4. Central nervous system tumours

Degenerative and metabolic disorders
1. Ganglioside storage diseases
2. Adrenoleukodystrophy
3. Neuronal ceroid lipofuscinoses
4. Organic acidurias
5. Mitochondrial encephalopathies
6. Gray-matter degenerative disorders

Developmental malformations
1. Anencephaly
2. Hydranencephaly
3. Lissencephaly
4. Holoprosencephaly
5. Encephaloceles
6. Schizencephaly
7. Congenital hydrocephalus
8. Severe microencephaly

From Ashwal (28) with permission.

In an extensive review of children in the vegetative state, Ashwal maintained that the diagnosis could not be reliably made under the age of 3 months, except in the anencephalic infant, because of the difficulty in distinguishing between voluntary and reflex behaviours in early infancy (28). The Task Force took the same view. Yet the Child Neurologists' survey recorded 20% of cases as less than 2 months of age (11). Ashwal maintained that children were more resistant to acute brain insults than adults (28) and he estimated the risk that various severe insults would result in the vegetative state, based on published cases (Table 3.17). He also listed the causes of the vegetative state in children, including the various degenerative, metabolic disorders and developmental malformations (Table 3.18).

REFERENCES

1 Ashwal S, Eyman RK, Call TL. Life expectancy of children in a persistent vegetative state. *Pediatr Neurol* 1994; 10: 27–33

2 Bricolo A, Turazzi S, Feriotti G. Prolonged posttraumatic unconsciousness *J Neurosurg* 1980; 52: 625–34

3 Minderhoud JM, Braakman R. Het vegeternde bestaan. *Ned Tijdschr Geneeskd* 1985; 129: 2385–8

4 Higashi K, Sakata Y, Hatano M et al. Epidemiological studies on patients with a persistent vegetative state. *J Neurol Neurosurg Psychiatry* 1977; 40: 870–78

5 Sato S, Imamura H, Ueki K et al. Epidemiological survey of vegetative state patients in the Tokohu District, Japan. *Neurol Med Chir (Tokyo)* 1978; 19: 141–5

6 Kitamura K, Morioka T, Fukui M et al. Patients with profoundly disturbed consciousness in Kyushu and Okinawa. In Hori S, Kanno T, Eds, *Proceeding of the 8ʰ Annual Meeting of The Society for Treatment of Coma*. Tokyo, Neuron, 1999: 3–16

7 Hellema H. 'Life termination' in the Netherlands. *BMJ* 1991; 302: 984–5

8 Tasseau F, Boucard MH, Le Gall JR et al. *États vegetative chroniques. Repercussions humaine aspects mediaux juridiques et éthiques*. Remmes: Éditions École Nationale de La Sante Publique, 1991

9 Tresch DD, Sims FH, Duthie EH et al. Clinical characteristics of patients in the persistent vegetative state. *Arch Intern Med* 1991; 151: 930–32

10 Spudis EV. The persistent vegetative state – 1990. *J Neurol Sci* 1991; 102: 128–36

11 Ashwal S, Bale JF, Coulter DL et al. The persistent vegetative state in children. Report of the Child Neurology Society Ethics Committee. *Ann Neurol* 1992; 32: 570–76

12 American Medical Association Council on Scientific Affairs and Council of Ethical and Judicial Affairs. Persistent vegetative state and the decision to withdraw or withhold life support. *JAMA* 1990; 263: 426–30

13 The Multi-Society Task Force on the Persistent Vegetative State. Statement on medical aspects of the persistent vegetative state. *N Engl J Med* 1994; 330: 1499–1508

14 Braakman R, Jennett B, Minderhoud JM. Prognosis of the posttraumatic vegetative state. *Acta Neurochir (Wien)* 1988; 95: 49–52

15 Murray LS, Teasdale GM, Murray GD et al. Does prediction of outcome alter patient management? *Lancet* 1993; 341: 1487–91

16 Marshall LF, Gautille T, Klauber MR et al. The outcome of severe closed head injury. *J Neurosurg* 1991; 25: S28–36

17 Sazbon L, Groswasser Z. Severe traumatic brain injury. *J Neurosurg* 1990; 73: 479–80

18 Murray GD, Teasdale GM, Braakman R et al. The European Brain Injury Consortium (EBIC) Survey of Head Injuries. *Acta Neurochir (Wien)* 1999; 141: 223–36

19 Levy DE, Bates D, Caronna JJ et al. Prognosis in non-traumatic coma. *Ann Intern Med* 1981; 94: 293–301

20 Cole G, Boyd S, Kendall B et al. Children in a persistent vegetative state *BMJ* 1984; 289: 1620–21

21 Jennett B. Some international comparisons. In: *Mild Head Injury*. Levin HS, Eisenberg HM, Benton AL (Eds). New York: Oxford University Press 1989: 23–34

22 Jennett B. Epidemiology of head injury. *J Neurol Neurosurg Psychiatry* 1996; 60: 362–9

23 Sazbon L, Costeff H, Groswasser Z. Epidemiological findings in traumatic post-comatose unawareness. *Brain Injury* 1992; 6: 359–62

24 Walshe TM, Leonard C. Persistent vegetative state. Extension of the syndrome to include chronic disorders. *Arch Neurol* 1985; 42: 1045–7

25 Volicer L, Berman SA, Cipolloni PB et al. Persistent vegetative state in Alzheimer disease: Does it exist? *Arch Neurol* 1997; 54: 1382–4

26 Gillies JD, Seshia SS. Vegetative state following coma in childhood: evolution and outcome. *Dev Med Child Neurol* 1980; 22: 642–8

27 Campbell AGM. Children in a persistent vegetative state. *BMJ* 1984; 289: 1022–3

28 Ashwal S. The persistent vegetative state in children. In: *Advances in Pediatrics* Vol 41. Barness LA (Ed). Mosby Year Book Inc 1994: 195–222

4

Pathology of the brain damage

Before the description of the vegetative state there were occasional reports of the structural damage in the brains of patients whom we would now probably call vegetative, and there have been a few since then. Reports up to 1994 were reviewed by Kinney and Samuels (1), although they included some traumatic cases who were not vegetative by the present definition. In hypoxic–ischaemic cases the damage is usually extensive necrosis in the cerebral cortex, almost always associated with thalamic damage. This is because of the selective vulnerability to hypoxia of the grey matter in the cerebral hemispheres. Occasionally, however, there is relative sparing of the cortex, with the main damage in the thalamus (2,3,4).

In traumatic cases the dominant lesion is diffuse damage to the subcortical white matter – what is now known as diffuse axonal injury (DAI). The original description of this type of brain damage was by Strich in 1956 and 1961 (5,6), when she proposed that this damage was the result of shearing forces acting on nerve fibres in the white matter of the cerebral hemispheres at the moment of injury. However, some continental European reports of these lesions in apallic patients claimed that this axonal damage was secondary to hypoxia and ischaemia related to high intracranial pressure (7,8,9). Such secondary intracranial complications are certainly common but experimental studies in nonhuman primates have subsequently shown that axonal damage identical to that found after head injury in humans can be produced as a primary lesion by nonimpact angular acceleration of the head without secondary hypoxia or ischaemia having occurred (10,11). It was these experimental studies and parallel clinical investigations that led Adams et al. (10) to introduce the term DAI, and they later defined three grades of severity of this lesion in humans (12). In the most severe (grade 3) there are, in addition to widespread damage to axons in all parts of the brain, focal lesions in the corpus callosum and in the dorsolateral sector of the rostral brain stem. In grade 2 DAI there is a focal lesion only in the corpus callosum, whilst in grade 1 there are no focal lesions – only the diffuse damage to axons. These focal lesions can often be seen at postmortem with the naked eye but sometimes microscopy is needed, as it always is for identifying the axonal injury. In earlier studies, the recognition of axonal injury depended on silver staining techniques but immunohistological methodology now makes for more reliable identification of this lesion (13,14).

The most detailed account of the pathological substrate of the vegetative state is a comparison of 35 traumatic cases with 14 of nontraumatic origin by Adams et al. (15). All had survived for at least a month since the brain insult, some for years. In the traumatic cases there was grade 2 or 3 DAI in 71%, and three others had grade 1 lesions. Of these three and the ten without any DAI all but one had moderate or severe ischaemic brain damage affecting the cerebral cortex or the thalamus or both. Altogether there was ischaemic brain damage in 43% of traumatic cases, related either to high intracranial pressure or to major extracranial injuries associated with systemic hypotension and/or hypoxia. The ischaemic cortical damage was diffuse in four and focal in nine cases. The cerebral cortex was completely normal in seven cases and in 21 others was affected only by minor traumatic contusions. The thalamus was abnormal in 80% of traumatic cases, diffusely so in 71%. Diffuse thalamic damage was often due to transneuronal degeneration from DAI, a lesion that cannot be recognized until some 3 months after injury; of those who survived this long, 96% had thalamic damage. Ischaemia accounted for the thalamic damage in cases without DAI. Only 14% of the traumatic cases had brain-stem damage, always slight and never haemorrhagic.

The pathological features of these 35 post-traumatic vegetative cases have been compared with those found in 30 brains of head injured patients who had recovered to a state of severe disability before death (16). Of the brains from the severely disabled, half had neither severe DAI nor thalamic damage, a negative combination not found in a single vegetative case. However, of the severely disabled, 20% had severe DAI, 37% had thalamic lesions and 7% had both. That some severely disabled patients had similar types of brain damage to that found in vegetative cases is probably explained by this damage being more severe in the vegetative cases. These studies have so far been focused on identifying the location and nature of the brain damage but have not been able to quantify this beyond classifying it as mild, moderate and severe.

Of the 14 nontraumatic cases seven had had a cardiac arrest, four an episode of arterial hypotension, and one each of asphyxia, smoke inhalation and intracranial infection. The most common abnormality in these nontraumatic cases was diffuse damage in the neocortex (64%). This took the form of laminar necrosis, with the damage increasing in intensity from the frontal to the occipital cortex. In three other cases cortical damage was restricted to arterial boundary zones, and in another affected more than one arterial territory. The only case with a normal neocortex was a case of asphyxia in which carbon monoxide may have played a part. As well as thalamic damage this brain had extensive damage to the subcortical white matter of a type associated with carbon monoxide poisoning (17,18). In every one of these nontraumatic cases there was profound diffuse neuronal loss in the thalamus and hippocampus. In eight of the 14 nontraumatic cases there were minor abnormalities in the brain stem.

After both severe DAI and severe cortical necrosis there is progressive Wallerian-type demyelination of the subcortical white matter and the descending tracts in the brain stem. With increasing duration of survival there is, consequently, progressive atrophy of the brain with *ex vacuo* hydrocephalus. In this series the brain weight was more than 500 g below normal in one traumatic and one nontraumatic case; two reported nontraumatic cases had weight losses of more than 400 g (3,19). This compares with about 200 g loss of weight in the brains of victims of the most advanced Alzheimer's disease.

The features common to all the cases in this series was diffuse damage to the white matter of the cerebral hemispheres and/or the thalamus. The cerebral cortex was undamaged in many traumatic cases and in occasional nontraumatic ones. Even in hypoxic cases the cortical damage was often patchy in distribution and the thalamic damage was then often dominant. Thalamic damage was found in all nontraumatic and most traumatic cases in this series. Kinney et al. (1) explain the vital role of the thalamus as a critical component of distributed neuronal networks underlying various cognitive and affective functions. They suggest that the thalamus provides, in a sense, a compact version of the cerebral cortex confined to a small locus and vascular supply; it is therefore very vulnerable to damage that can disrupt much cortical function. One traumatic vegetative case investigated by Schiff et al. (20) had normal metabolic activity in most of the cortex, the damage being limited to the thalamus. These authors also reported the persistence in a few vegetative patients of some complex behaviours that may involve limited cortical circuits associated with islands of preserved metabolic cortical activity (p. 17). The finding of only patchy cortical damage at autopsy in some cases is consistent with these findings in living patients. The presumption is that, in spite of some cortical sparing there is in the vegetative state insufficient cortex surviving or adequately connected to other cortical areas, either directly or via the thalamus, for cognitive activity and awareness.

REFERENCES

1 Kinney HC, Samuels MA. Neuropathology of the persistent vegetative state – a review. *J Neuropathol Exp Neurol* 1994; 53: 548–58

2 Relkin NR, Petito CK, Plum F. Coma and the vegetative state associated with thalamic injury after cardiac arrest. *Ann Neurol* 1990; 28: 221

3 Kinney HC, Korein J, Panigaphy A et al. Neuropathological findings in the brain of Karen Ann Quinlan. The role of the thalamus in the persistent vegetative state. *N Eng J Med* 1994; 330: 1469–75

4 Jellinger K. The brain of Karen Ann Quinlan (letter). *N Eng J Med* 1994; 331: 1378–9

5 Strich SJ. Diffuse degeneration of cerebral white matter and severe dementia following head injury. *J Neurol Neurosurg Psychiatry* 1956; 19: 163–85

6 Strich SJ. Shearing of nerve fibres as a cause of brain damage due to head injury. *Lancet* 1961; 2: 444–8

7 Jellinger K, Seitelberger F. Protracted post-traumatic encephalopathy: pathology, pathogenesis and clinical implications. *J Neurol Sci* 1970; 10: 51–94

8 Jellinger K. Pathology and pathogenesis of apallic syndromes following closed head injuries. In Ore GD, Gerstenbrand F, Lucking CH et al. (Eds). *The Apallic Syndrome.* Berlin: Springer-Verlag. 1977: 88–103

9 Peters G, Rothemund NB. Neuropathology of the traumatic apallic syndrome. In Ore GD, Gerstenbrand F, Lucking CH et al. (Eds). *The Apallic Syndrome.* Berlin: Springer-Verlag. 1977: 78–87

10 Adams JH, Graham DI, Murray LS et al. Diffuse axonal injury due to nonmissile head injury in humans: an analysis of 45 cases. *Ann Neurol* 1982; 12: 557–63

11 Gennarelli TA, Thibault LE, Adams JH et al. Diffuse axonal injury and traumatic coma in the primate. *Ann Neurol* 1982; 12: 564–74

12 Adams JH, Doyle D. Ford I et al. Diffuse axonal injury: definition, diagnosis and grading. *Histopathology* 1989; 15: 40–59

13 Gentleman SM, Nash MJ, Sweeting CJ et al. β-Amyloid precursor protein (BAPP) as a marker for axonal injury after head injury. *Neurosci Lett* 1963; 160: 139–44

14 Sherriff FE, Bridges LR, Sivaloganathan S. Early detection of axonal injury after

human head trauma using immunocytochemistry for β-amyloid presursor protein. *Acta Neuropath* 1944; 87: 55–62

15 Adams JE, Graham DI, Jennett B. The neuropathology of the vegetative state after an acute brain insult. *Brain* 2000; 123: 1327–38

16 Jennett B, Adams JH, Murray LS et al. Neuropathology in vegetative and severely disabled patients after head injury. *Ann Neurol* 2001; 56: 486–90

17 Lapresle J, Fardeau M. The leukoencephalopathies caused by carbon monoxide poisoning; study of 16 anatomo-clinical observations *Acta Neuropathol (Berl)* 1966; 6: 327–48

18 Hart IK, Kennedy PG, Adams JH et al. Neurological manifestations of carbon monoxide poisoning. *Postgrad Med J* 1988; 64: 213–16

19 Cole G, Cowie VA. Long survival after cardiac arrest: case report and neuropathological findings. *Clin Neuropathol* 1987; 6: 104–5

20 Schiff N, Ribary U, Moreno D et al. Residual cerebral activity and behavioral fragments can remain in the persistently vegetative state. *Brain.* In press

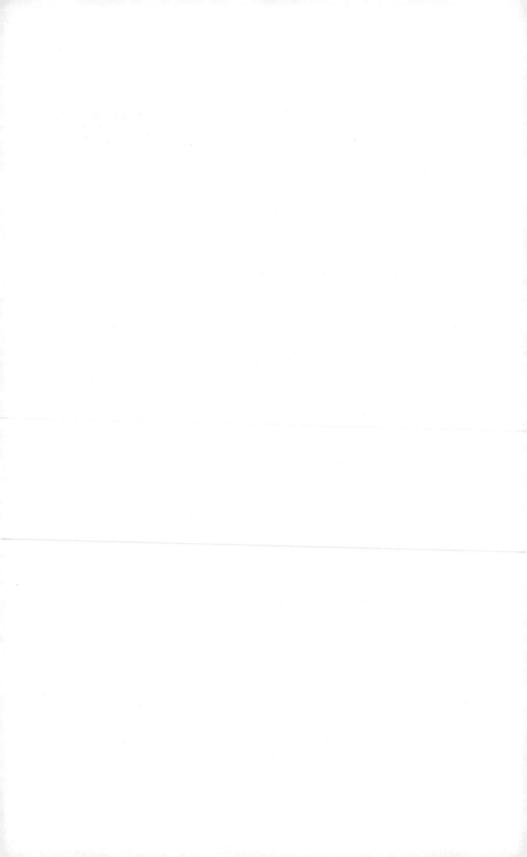

5

Prognosis for recovery and survival

The original description of the persistent vegetative state was careful to note that no data were then available to indicate how long this state must persist before it can be declared permanent. Since then there have been a number of published reports, the analysis of which led the US Task Force in 1994 (1) to publish tables that are now widely accepted as a basis for decision making by both the medical and legal professions. Before considering these it is important to consider how data on outcome has accumulated over the years and has informed various prognostic statements before the Task Force paper.

Data on recovery

In a follow-up for 1–7 years of 62 patients who had been completely apallic after head injury, Pagni et al. (2) reported in 1977 that 38 were dead, ten severely disabled and nine independent. In 1978, Levy et al. (3) reported on the follow-up of 25 patients who had been vegetative 1 month after nontraumatic coma. By the end of a year only two had uttered any words but neither had obeyed commands; by then one of these two and 17 others had died. In 1980, Bricolo et al. (4) reported 135 cases who were unconsciousness for at least 2 weeks after head injury, of whom 102 had eye opening at 1 month. By 3 months, 52% were obeying commands, with an additional 13% doing so by 6 months, and 1.5% more by 12 months. The conclusion was that recovery from the vegetative state could occur up to a year after head injury. In 1985, Sazbon (5) reported 173 patients vegetative at one month, 32% of them after nontraumatic insults. By 6 months 47% of the traumatic and 21% of the nontraumatic had regained consciousness; by 1 year only 4% more of the traumatic cases and none of the nontraumatic had recovered. Of the traumatic cases twice as many who were under

Table 5.1. One year outcomes of patients in VS after head injury

Duration of VS	n	Dead (%)	Vegetative (%)	Conscious[a] (%)	Independent (%)
1 month	140	51	11	36	10
3 months	49	49	31	20	0
6 months	30	32	52	16	0

[a]Includes independent.
Data from Braakman et al. (7).

Table 5.2. Independence at 1 year from patients in VS 1 month after head injury

Age	n	% independent
<20 years	53	21
20–39 years	46	9
>40 years	41	0

Data from Braakman et al. (7).

the age of 45 years had recovered as in the older group. In 1986, Berrol (6) summarized some of the above reports together with data on traumatic cases later published by Braakman et al. (7). He added that not one of 20 rehabilitation physicians questioned had seen recovery to independence after 6 months in a traumatic vegetative state, and that none would persist with intensive therapy for more than a year.

The study of Braakman et al. (7) in 1988 analysed 140 patients vegetative 1 month after head injury. After a year, 51% were dead, 11% vegetative, 26% severely disabled and 10% had become independent. Of those still vegetative at 3 and 6 months, none became independent; the longer they were vegetative the fewer became conscious and the more remained vegetative by the end of a year (Table 5.1). Recovery to independence was twice as frequent in patients under 20 years of age as in those aged 20–39 years; no one over 40 recovered this well (Table 5.2).

The first institutional pronouncement on prognosis was the 1989 Position Statement from the American Academy of Neurology (8). Its main focus was on the acceptability of withdrawing artificial nutrition and hydration once the vegetative state was deemed to be permanent. It stated that permanent unconsciousness could usually be diagnosed with a high degree of medical certainty 1–3 months after a hypoxic–ischaemic brain insult. No reference was made to data supporting this assertion either in the statement or in the accompanying commentary (9). Nor was any mention made about the prognosis after traumatic insults – although several series of such cases had by then been published.

The following year came the report from the Council on Scientific Affairs of the American Medical Association, based on the scientific literature up to June 1989 (10). It concluded that of those vegetative for 1 month after asphyxial injury few if any regained cognition, and after 3 months essentially none did. Permanence after trauma could be assumed after 1 year, but for head-injured patients over 50 years recovery was vanishingly rare after 6 months. Taking account of two reported cases of later recovery than this (11,12) the odds of recovery using these recommended criteria for permanence were estimated at less than 1 in 1000.

The Traumatic Coma Data Bank in 1991 reported the follow-up of 93 adults who were vegetative on discharge (13). Because the median hospital stay for these patients was 59 days and some left the acute hospital as soon as 5 days after injury, this series was likely to have included some patients who were vegetative for less than a month. Not all were followed for a year but of those followed for at least 6 months, 58% regained consciousness and 8% became independent. Although six patients were claimed to have regained consciousness after 1 year, some doubt has arisen about the validity of this observation (p. 63).

The largest series followed for 1 year was reported from France in 1994 by Danze et al. (14). Of 522 who were vegetative 1 month after head injury (16% of them under 20 years of age), 61% had regained consciousness at the end of a year, with 14% having become independent. One year mortality increased steadily with age from 4% for below 20 years to 49% for 60 years and over. Fewer of the adult patients became independent (5%) than of the under 20s (24%).

Task Force data

The Multi-Society Task Force comprised adult and paediatric neurologists and neurosurgeons, representing five major medical societies in the US, all of which approved the final statement. Its report in 1994 therefore carried great authority (1). Its conclusions about prognosis were based on review of 754 cases published in the English language literature who were

Table 5.3. One-year outcome of those in VS at 1 month

Age	n	Dead (%)	Vegetative (%)	Conscious[a] (%)	Independent (%)
Traumatic					
Adults	434	33	15	52	24
Children	106	9	29	62	27
Nontraumatic					
Adults	169	53	32	15	4
Children	45	22	65	13	6

[a] Includes independent.
Data from Task Force (1).

vegetative at 1 month after an acute insult and for whom 1 year outcome was available. Emphasis was put on the difference between recovery of consciousness and of function because, although some patients regain their independence, most who are recorded as having 'recovered' after months in the vegetative state remain very severely disabled and totally dependent. The data on outcome was given separately for traumatic and nontraumatic cases, and for adults and children (age limit not defined but most were probably under 16 years). The recovery pattern at 12 months after insult of those vegetative at 1 month revealed that nontraumatic cases less often recovered (Table 5.3). Among these nontraumatic cases the hypoxic cases did worse than the others. Children did somewhat better, especially after head injury. Of the whole series, 43% regained consciousness, ranging from 62% for head injured children to 13% for nontraumatic children. Only 19% of all cases became independent (6% good recovery and 13% moderate disability on the Glasgow Outcome Scale). The highest independent rate was in head injured children (27%), the lowest in nontraumatic adults (4%).

With such a substantial recovery rate for patients vegetative a month after acute brain damage, some guarded optimism is justified during the first 3 months. For later decision making it is important to know the prognosis of patients who are still vegetative after 3, 6 and 12 months. The Task Force calculated the probability of various outcomes after 3 and 6 months in a vegetative state by age and cause (Tables 5.4 and 5.5). The numbers in some cells are small, so that the 99% confidence intervals are

Table 5.4. Probability of 1-year outcomes for those in VS for 3 months

Age	n	Dead (%)	Vegetative (%)	Conscious[a] (%)	Independent (%)
Traumatic					
Adults	218	35 (27–43)	30 (22–38)	35 (27–44)	16 (10–22)
Children	50	14 (1–27)	30 (13–47)	56 (37–74)	32 (15–49)
Nontraumatic					
Adults	77	46 (31–61)	47 (32–62)	8 (2–19)	1 (0–4)
Children	31	3 (0–11)	94 (83–100)	3 (0–11)	0

Figures in parentheses are 99% confidence limits.
[a]Includes independent.
Data from Task Force (1).

Table 5.5. Probabilities of 1-year outcomes for those in VS for 6 months

Age	n	Dead (%)	Vegetative (%)	Conscious[a] (%)	Independent (%)
Traumatic					
Adults	123	32 (21–43)	52 (40–64)	16 (9–27)	4 (0–9)
Children	28	14 (0–31)	54 (30–78)	32 (12–58)	11 (0–26)
Nontraumatic					
Adults	50	28 (12–44)	72 (56–88)	0	0
Children	30	0	97 (89–100)	3 (0–11)	0

Figures in parentheses are 99% confidence limits.
[a]Includes independent.
Data from Task Force (1).

wide. From the data published, an alternative analysis shows the prognosis for each cause regardless of age, by age for both causes together, and for the whole series (Tables 5.6–5.9). Previous studies had shown that older adults have less chance of recovery of consciousness and of independence. The Task Force concluded from analysis of the 754 cases reviewed that the vegetative state could reasonably be declared permanent 3 months after nontraumatic damage and 12 months after head injury in both children and adults. However, when over 300 American physicians were questioned a year before the Task Force report, many had felt able to declare the vegetative state permanent after their patients had been vegetative for only

Table 5.6. Dead (%) at 1 year of those in VS at 1, 3 and 6 months
(*n* at 1 month)

	Adults (*n* = 603)	Children (*n* = 151)	Trauma (*n* = 540)	Nontrauma (*n* = 214)	All (*n* = 754)
1 month	39	13	28	47	34
3 months	38	10	31	36	32
6 months	31	7	28	18	25

Data from Task Force (1).

Table 5.7. Conscious (%) at 1 year of those in VS at 1, 3 and 6 months
(*n* at 1 month)

	Adults (*n* = 603)	Children (*n* = 151)	Trauma (*n* = 540)	Nontrauma (*n* = 214)	All (*n* = 754)
1 month	42	48	54	14	43
3 months	27	36	39	6	30
6 months	12	17	19	1	13

Data from Task Force (1).

Table 5.8. Independent (%) at 1 year of those in VS at 1, 3 and 6 months
(*n* at 1 month)

	Adults (*n* = 603)	Children (*n* = 151)	Trauma (*n* = 540)	Nontrauma (*n* = 214)	All (*n* = 754)
1 month	18	21	25	5	19
3 months	12	20	19	1	14
6 months	3	5	5	0	4

Data from Task Force (1).

4–8 weeks after a hypoxic incident, and for 8–10 weeks after a head injury (15). In the European study of over 2000 doctors in seven countries a year after the Task Force report, 17% were very or quite confident of the ultimate outcome in less than 3 months, and 38% were by 4–6 months (16).

Table 5.9. Vegetative (%) at 1 year of those in VS at 1, 3 and 6 months
(*n* at 1 month)

	Adults (*n* = 603)	Children (*n* = 151)	Trauma (*n* = 540)	Nontrauma (*n* = 214)	All (*n* = 754)
1 month	19	39	18	39	23
3 months	35	54	30	58	38
6 months	57	76	53	81	62

Data from Task Force (1).

Late recoveries

The Task Force recognized that there were occasional single case reports of limited recovery beyond these periods and that its recommendations were based on probabilities, and that they represented only 'reasonable medical certainty' that further recovery was very unlikely. The Task Force reviewed 30 media reports alleging unexpected recovery from prolonged coma or vegetative survival (personal communication). It found that in 15 of these cases awareness had in fact recovered before the recommended period for declaring permanence. From the limited information available about the others, the impression was that only two had definitely been vegetative (each recovered 5 months after a nontraumatic insult). Another four had possibly been vegetative, and the remaining nine certainly not. The titles of some reports in the medical literature can be misleading. Two papers claiming recovery after prolonged postanoxic vegetative state (17) and after prolonged hypoxic coma (18) in fact reported recoveries after only 7 and 8 weeks. Another 'unexpected' recovery was at 10 months after head injury (19).

Of more interest are the medically verified recoveries that had begun outside the limits for determining permanence. The Task Force review included 214 nontraumatic cases followed for 1 year (i.e. for 9 months beyond the permanence period), but no substantial traumatic series has been followed after 1 year. The Traumatic Data Bank followed 25 cases for 1–3 years and initially claimed that six had regained consciousness during this period (13). However, follow-up had been only by telephone and it has since been discovered that three of these six had improved before 1 year and there are no clinical details of the remaining three, according to Childs

Table 5.10. Late recoveries
(> 3 months nontraumatic, > 12 months traumatic)

Author (ref)	Year	Age	Cause	Months in VS
Rosenberg (21)	1977	43	Anoxia	17
Higashi (22)	1981	26	Anoxia	8
Higashi (22)	1981	61	SAH	36
Snyder (12)	1983	36	Anoxia	22
Arts (11)	1985	18	HI	30
Andrews (23)	1993	27	Anoxia	4
Andrews (23)	1993	42	Anoxia	11
Andrews (23)	1993	20	Anoxia	6
Andrews (23)	1993	47	Anoxia	6
Childs (20)	1996	18	HI	15
Dyer (24)	1997	22	Anoxia	84

SAH, subarachnoid haemorrhage; HI, head injury.

et al. (20). They commented that the Task Force had accepted a 1.6% possible error rate for declaring permanence, but if the three cases above are accepted, then for that study the error rate would be 3/22 (14%). For the most part, reports of late recoveries depend on single case reports of which five were tabulated by the Task Force, but it acknowledged four other cases. These nine cases and two more recent ones are set out in Table 5.10. Some alleged late recoveries might in fact have been late discoveries of earlier recovery. Given the interest in late recoveries provoked by the time limits proposed by the Task Force for declaring permanence, it might have been expected that most exceptions to these since then would have been reported, but only two have been. What is clear is that these late recoveries are almost always to very severe disability. Most patients remain totally dependent, some reaching only the minimally conscious state or a little better. Many continue to require tube feeding and are able to communicate only by gesture or coded movements because they cannot speak.

Prediction of recovery

As the weeks pass and the patient remains vegetative there is increasing pressure on doctors to make some estimate of the chances of the return of consciousness and of useful function. For the two main causes and for adults and children the Task Force probabilities can give some indication of the likelihood of recovery. For adults it seems from several studies that increasing age reduces the chances of recovery of consciousness and of function, whilst within nontraumatic cases those with anoxic damage appear to do less well. Yet most of the reported cases of late recovery have been among those with anoxic brain damage. Some vegetative patients show more reflex activity than others do and it is natural to expect that those who are more active might have a better prognosis – but no such correlation was found by Higashi et al. (25). Because the return of visual pursuit and/or a blink response to visual threat are often the first signs of recovery the presence of either does suggest a better than average chance of recovery. However, such behaviours have been observed in some patients who then remained vegetative in every other respect for many years. Few features of predictive value were found in a statistical analysis of a large series of traumatic cases in France (14). More recoveries occurred when there was a blink to threat, and fewer when imaging showed marked hydrocephalus. Whether or not diffuse axonal injury was demonstrated by imaging did not affect prognosis. This was at variance with a German study that found that vegetative patients who regained consciousness at 1 year had less evidence of DAI on MRI at 6 weeks after injury than those who remained vegetative (26). However, there was DAI in a quarter of the recovered cases so that this finding was not a reliable predictor – and pathological studies bear this out (p. 52). Two cases of late recovery frequently referred to had shown only a little ventricular dilatation on late CT scans (11,12), so that lack of marked and progressive hydrocephalus probably does indicate an above average potential for recovery.

Expectation of life

For most patients vegetative at 1 month after an acute brain insult there is a high mortality in the first year, by which time a third of the Task Force patients were dead. However, there was considerable variation between different patient groups, ranging from 9% for head-injured children to 53% for nontraumatic adults (Table 5.11). Different authors also report a range of early mortality figures – from 19% (14) to 51% (7) for head-injured patients. Fewer data are available on long-term mortality but it is

Table 5.11. One-year mortality for patients in VS at 1 month

Reference	Case type	n	Dead (%)
Task Force (1)	All	754	34
	Adults	603	39
	Children	151	13
	Trauma	540	28
	Nontrauma	214	47
	Nontrauma adults	169	53
	Trauma children	106	9
Danze et al. (14)	Trauma	522	19
Sazbon (5)	Trauma	117	31
	Nontrauma	56	59
Braakman et al. (7)	Trauma	140	51

Table 5.12. Late mortality

		Percentage of n			
Reference	n	3 years	5 years	6 years	8 years
In VS at 1 month					
Task Force adults (27)	603	70	84		
Higashi et al. (25)	110	65	73		
In VS at 6 months					
Minderhoud et al. (28)	53	47		76	78

evident that in those who survive for several years the continuing mortality is low (Table 5.12). Mean survival after acute damage in the Task Force review ranged from 2 to 5 years (1). In a small series of those vegetative from chronic dementing conditions, mean survivals ranged from 3.5 to 7 years, with some surviving 16 years (29).

The question of long-term survival is a matter of some debate that particularly concerns health providers and litigation lawyers because of the large cost implications of providing total care for many years (30). Occasional reports appear of exceptionally long survivals, such as those of 18 years (31), 37 years (32) and 41 years (33). Whilst acknowledging such reports, the Task Force concluded that survival beyond 10 years was unusual. Yet, following a British TV documentary on the vegetative state in

1994, responses to a telephone help line logged 458 members of the public related to vegetative family members, 78 of whom had been in VS for more than 10 years (34). There have been other reports of more than 20 years survival (28,35). The Task Force calculated that for those vegetative at 1 month the probability of survival for more than 15 years was very low (less than 1 in 15 000–75 000). However, predictions of long-term survival are of most interest in those who have already survived a year or more in a vegetative state. By this time, many have recovered and others have died so that less than a quarter of all patients and less than a fifth of traumatic cases who were vegetative at 1 month are by then still vegetative (Table 5.9). This means that the estimated probabilities of long survival based on patients vegetative after only 1 month should be increased in those who have survived the first year by 4 times for all cases and by 5 times for traumatic cases. Indeed, it is the experience of clinicians dealing with long-term care that, once the first year is survived, many vegetative patients become quite stable, and data on late mortality support this (Table 5.12). Immediately following the Task Force report there were letters protesting that their estimates of long-term survival were too low (36,37), and pointing out that many reported deaths might have been the result of decisions to limit treatment. There might therefore be a difference between how long such patients **could** live and how long they **do** live, and this may become more significant as the practice of limiting treatment once a vegetative state is declared permanent becomes more widely accepted. Some rehabilitation-ists have claimed, however, that long survival might become more common with modern methods of care, yet, by definition, the long-term survivors already reported have not benefited from this; indeed, some reports have emphasized that the care of a long survivor had been in an unsophisticated institution.

In contrast to these anecdotal reports, some systematic studies have emerged from a paediatrician and statistician in California. In 1992, a questionnaire to child neurologists revealed that duration of survival varied according to age, from 4.1 to 7.4 years (Table 5.13). A further study of an actual series by Ashwal et al. (39) found similar figures, although it seems curious that 150 patients of 19 years and older were classified as children (Table 5.14). A more recent report dealt with patients who had suffered a head injury between the ages of 5 and 21 years and who were left with various degrees of disability, 23% of whom were followed for 5 years or more (40). The 21 vegetative patients were not dealt with separately as

Table 5.13. Mean survival of children in VS

Age	Years survival
<2 months	4.1
2 months–2 years	5.5
2–7 years	7.3
7–18 years	7.4

Child Neurologists' estimates, Ashwal et al. (38).

Table 5.14. Survival of 847 PVS children in VS

	n	Median (years)
Age		
<1 year	193	2.6
1–2 years	112	4.2
3–6 years	191	5.2
7–18 years	201	7.0
>19 years	150	9.9
Etiology		
Trauma	124	3.0
Nontraumatic	138	8.8
Infection	87	2.6
Perinatal	150	4.1
Chromosomal/ Developmental	110	8.2
Miscellaneous	238	6.7

From Ashwal et al. (39).

they were found not to differ in life expectation from the 109 others who were also immobile and tube fed 6 months after injury. For such patients at age 15 years, the remaining life expectancy for males was estimated as 15 years, compared with a normal of 58 years. A further study involved over 1000 vegetative patients and was limited to those who had already survived in this state for 1 year (41). The mortality rate fell by 8% for each extra year of survival between 1 and 10 years in the vegetative state, so that after 7 years survival the future mortality was only 60% of what it had been after 1 year in the vegetative state. This study also drew attention to the difference between the **mean** expectation of life and the **median** survival time (by which time half of the patients will have died). It is the latter that concerns lawyers in civil courts working to the 'more probable than not' standard of proof. This is always a shorter time than the mean. For example, 15-year-olds who have been vegetative for one year have a mean expectation of 10.5 years but a median survival time of only 5.2 years; if still vegetative after 4 years, these figures are 12.2 years and 7 years, respectively. About half the patients in this study were tube fed and this feature increased the mortality by 2.5 times. No secular trend towards lower mortality was found over the period 1981 to 1996 for those aged 10–30 years (when 1-year-vegetative), but there had been an improvement for younger children. However, surveys in Japan, mostly of older adults with nontraumatic causes, found that, while only 15% of vegetative patients lived more than 3 years in 1975, 35% did so in 1997 (42).

A study of a large number of children aged 3–15 years compared the life expectancy of those who were vegetative and those who were minimally conscious (43). The definition of the latter was probably not as rigorous as has been recommended recently (p. 24). Indeed many of the minimally conscious had a degree of mobility, defined as one or more of these actions: ability to lift the head when lying prone, to lift a limb, to roll over or to sit unaided for 5 minutes (less than 10% could do this last task). Survival for 8 years for the **immobile** minimally conscious was similar to that of the vegetative group (65% and 63%, respectively) but it was significantly longer (81%) in the minimally conscious who were somewhat **mobile**. Many of these children had degenerative and genetic disorders and mortality was higher in them than in those with acquired brain damage. Only 37% of the vegetative and 12% of the minimally conscious had acquired brain damage, which was traumatic in 29%.

Cause of death

These were reviewed by the Task Force (1) in 143 patients. Pulmonary or urinary-tract infection accounted for 52%, systemic failure for 30%, sudden death for 9% and respiratory failure for 6%. If a patient has had recurrent infections, then a shorter expectation of life than average would be expected. Older patients are less likely to have very long survival, not only because of greater vulnerability to infections and other complications, but also because of the normal diseases of ageing – cardiovascular and cerebrovascular conditions and tumours – which accounted for 3% of deaths in the above series. The vegetative patient is unable to complain of the early symptoms of such conditions and so cannot benefit from timely treatment. Obviously, any progressive disease present before becoming vegetative will reduce the likelihood of prolonged survival.

REFERENCES

1 The Multi-Society Task Force on PVS: Medical aspects of the persistent vegetative state (part 2). *N Engl J Med* 1994; 330: 1572–9

2 Pagni CA, Giovanelli M, Tomei G et al. Long term results in 62 cases of post-traumatic complete apallic syndrome. *Acta Neurochir (Wien)* 1977; 36: 37–45

3 Levy DE, Knill-Jones RP, Plum F. The vegetative state and its prognosis following non-traumatic coma. *Ann N Y Acad Sci* 1978; 315: 293–306

4 Bricolo A, Turazzi S, Ferioti G. Prolonged post-traumatic unconsciousness. *J Neurosurg.* 1980; 52: 625–34

5 Sazbon L. Prolonged coma. *Progress in Clinical Neurosciences* 1985; 2: 65–81

6 Berrol S. Evolution and the persistent vegetative state. *J Head Trauma Rehabil* 1986; 1: 7–13

7 Braakman R, Jennett WB, Minderhoud JM. Prognosis of the posttraumatic vegetative state. *Acta Neurochir (Wien)* 1988; 95: 49–52

8 Executive Board, American Academy of Neurology. Position of the American Academy of Neurology on certain aspects of the care and management of the persistent vegetative state patient. *Neurology* 1989; 39: 125–6

9 Munsat TL, Stuart WH, Cranford RE. Guidelines on the vegetative state: Commentary on the American Academy of Neurology statement. *Neurology* 1989; 39: 123–4

10 Council on Scientific Affairs and Council on Ethical and Judicial Affairs of the American Medical Association. Persistent vegetative state and the decision to withdraw or withhold life support. *JAMA* 1990; 263: 426–30

11 Arts WFM, van Dongen HR, van Hof-van Duin J et al. Unexpected improvement after prolonged post-traumatic vegetative state. *J Neurol Neurosurg Psychiatry* 1985; 48: 1300–303

12 Snyder BD, Cranford RE, Rubens AB et al. Delayed recovery from postanoxic persistent vegetative state. *Ann Neurol* 1983; 14: 152

13 Levin HS, Saydjari C, Eisenberg HM et al. Vegetative state after closed head injury: A Traumatic Coma Data Bank report. *Arch Neurol* 1991; 48: 580–85

14 Danze F, Veys B, Lebrun T et al. Prognositic factors of post-traumatic vegetative states: 522 cases. *Neuro-Chirurgie* 1994; 40: 348–57

15 Payne K, Taylor RM, Stocking C et al. Physicians' attitudes about the care of

patients in the persistent vegetative state: a national survey. *Ann Intern Med* 1996; 125: 104–10

16 Grubb A, Walsh P, Lambe N et al. *The moral and legal issues surrounding the treatment and care of patients in persistent vegetative state.* Report to European Biomedical and Health Research Programme. 1997 [on file in the library of the Centre of Medical Law and Ethics, King's College London]

17 Shuttleworth E. Recovery to social and economic independence from prolonged postanoxic vegetative state. *Neurology* 1983; 33: 372–4

18 Falk RH. Physical and intellectual recovery following prolonged hypoxic coma. *Postgrad Med J* 1990; 66: 384–6

19 Jordan FM, Murdoch BE. Unexpected recovery of functional communication following a prolonged period of mutism post-head injury. *Brain Injury* 1990; 4: 101–8

20 Childs NL, Mercer WN. Brief report: Late improvement in consciousness after post-traumatic vegetative state. *N Engl J Med* 1996; 334: 24–5

21 Rosenberg GA, Johnson SF, Brenner RP. Recovery of cognition after prolonged vegetative state. *Ann Neurol.* 1977; 2: 167–8

22 Higashi K, Hatano M, Abiko S. Five year follow-up study of patients with a persistent vegetative state. *J Neurol Neurosurg Psychiatry* 1981; 44: 552–4

23 Andrews K. Recovery of patients after four months or more in the persistent vegetative state. *BMJ* 1993; 306: 1597–1600

24 Dyer C. Hillsborough survivor emerges from the permanent vegetative state. *BMJ* 1997; 314: 996

25 Higashi K, Sakata Y, Hatano M. Epidemiological studies on patients with a persistent vegetative state. *J Neurol Neurosurg Psychiatry* 1977; 40: 876–85

26 Kampfl A, Schmutzhard E, Franz G et al. Prediction of recovery from post-traumatic vegetative state. *Lancet* 1998; 351: 1763–7

27 Ashwal S, Cranford R. Multi-Society Task Force Report on PVS: correction on long-term survival data. *N Engl J Med* 1995; 333: 130

28 Minderhoud JM, Braakman R. Het vegeterende bestaan. *Ned Tijdschr Geneeskd* 1985; 129: 2385–8

29 Walshe TM, Leonard C. Persistent vegetative state: Extension of the syndrome to include chronic disorders. *Arch Neurol* 1985; 42: 1045–7

30 Paris JJ. The six-million-dollar woman. *Conn Med* 1981; 45: 720–21

31 Field RE, Romanus RJ. A decerebrate patient: eighteen years of care. *Conn Med* 1981; 45: 717–19

32 Cranford RE. Termination of treatment in the persistent vegetative state. *Semin Neurology* 1984; 4: 36–44

33 Sibbison JB. USA: right to live or right to die. *Lancet* 1991; 337: 102–3

34 Jennett B. A quarter century of the vegetative state: an international perspective. *J Head Trauma Rehabil* 1997; 12: 1–12

35 Wall M. Irish Supreme Court approves 'right to die' case. *Lancet* 1995; 346: 368

36   Haigh AJ. The persistent vegetative state (letter). *N Engl J Med* 1994; 331: 1380

37   Whyte J. The persistent vegetative state (letter). *N Engl J Med* 1994; 331: 1381

38   Ashwal S, Bale J, Coulter D et al. The persistent vegetative state in children: Report of the Child Neurology Society Ethics Committee. *Ann Neurol* 1992; 32: 570–76

39   Ashwal S, Eyman RK, Call TL. Life expectancy of children in the persistent vegetative state. *Pediatr Neurol* 1994; 10: 27–33

40   Strauss DJ, Shavelle RM, Anderson TW. Long-term survival of children and adolescents after traumatic brain injury. *Arch Phys Med Rehabil* 1998; 79: 1095–1100

41   Strauss DJ, Shavelle RM, Ashwal S. Life expectancy and median survival time in the permanent vegetative state. *Pediatr Neurol* 1999; 21: 626–31

42   Kitamura K, Morioka T, Fukui M et al. Patients with profoundly disturbed consciousness in Kyushu and Okinawa. In Hori S, Kanno T. (Eds). *Proceeding of the 8th Annual Meeting of The Society for Treatment of Coma.* Tokyo, Neuron, 1999: 3–16

43   Strauss DJ, Ashwal S, Day SM et al. Life expectancy of children in vegetative and minimally conscious states. *Pediatr Neurol* 2000; 23: 312–19

6

Attitudes to the permanent vegetative state

The medical, ethical, legal and public policy controversies that have followed the recognition of this state stem from how different people regard indefinite survival in a vegetative state. The arguments have focused mainly on the issue of withholding or withdrawing life-prolonging medical treatment, and later chapters deal with the ethical and legal issues raised by contemplating such a decision. However, the question of limiting treatment must be anticipated to some extent in this chapter because information about how the vegetative state is regarded comes partly from the comments of ethicists and lawyers dealing with this problem, as well as from asking various groups of people how they would themselves want to be treated if they were permanently vegetative, and professionals how they would want to deal with their vegetative patients.

In 1969, before the vegetative state was formally described, a physicist from Cambridge University wrote 'An appeal to doctors' in the *Lancet* (1). He imagined the horror of surviving after a road accident with severe brain damage (p. xii), and claimed that it was no longer generally true that it was always in a patient's interest that life should be preserved by all available means. The editorial response was unsympathetic but two years later, when the *Lancet* reported two patients who had survived for 5 months with neocortical necrosis from anoxic brain damage, an editorial comment was titled 'Death of a human being' (2). It asked whether anyone would actually want his own vegetative existence to be artificially prolonged and who that knows the facts would want a close relative so supported? In an address to the annual meeting of the British Medical Association in 1972, the Bishop of Durham in England questioned what degree of respect should be accorded to vegetative patients as compared with the lives of others who were much more evidently alive and in rapport with other members of society (3). The principle of respect for life, he said, had to be qualified and married to an explicit concept of personality and linked with ideas about the quality of life.

Table 6.1. Opinions about outcome of brain damage

Outcome	Audience (*n*)	For patient (%)	For family (%)
Vegetative worse than death	San Francisco experts (130)	87	96
	Glasgow students (130)	88	94
Severe disability worse than vegetative	San Francisco experts (130)	44	18
	Glasgow students (130)	41	14

From Jennett (4).

The first explicit reference to the vegetative state being regarded as worse than death was in 1976, when Jennett (4) reported the anonymous responses of two very different audiences to questions about this matter. One was 130 health professionals and lawyers attending a meeting on severe brain damage in San Francisco, the other a class of 130 medical students in their first year of clinical studies in Glasgow, Scotland. In spite of the contrasts between their ages, experience and cultural backgrounds their opinions were remarkably similar (Table 6.1). Nearly 90% considered that the vegetative state was worse than death, a few commenting that for the patient the question was irrelevant. Nearly 95% thought that families would consider it worse. More surprising, as this was more than 25 years ago, was that over 40% believed that very severe disability with dependence might be worse than being vegetative for the patients, but many fewer thought that families were likely to take this view. It was noted that subsequent surveys among nurses and general practitioners in Britain, and among nurses and students in the Netherlands, had shown similar responses. This report came in the same year that the *Quinlan* case about treatment withdrawal came to court in New Jersey (p. 127). In 1984 an American paediatrician titled his paper on the vegetative state in childhood 'A fate worse than death' (5), and a British paediatrician quoting this opined that any treatment that prolonged this 'non-human, artificial life' in a child was wrong (6). In 1987, *The Independent* newspaper in London headlined a whole page feature on a named vegetative patient 'A fate worse than death' – without a question mark (7).

The President's Commission in 1983 (8) concluded that the only value of prolonging the life of a permanently vegetative patient lay in the very remote chance of unexpected recovery. However, it noted that such late recoveries were followed by such severe disability as to be regarded by most patients as of very limited benefit, and that this was a major objection to continuing life support in the hope of late recovery. It referred with approval to several court cases that had allowed the withdrawal of life-sustaining treatment, including artificial nutrition and hydration (ANH). In 1986 the Council on Ethical and Judicial Affairs of the AMA declared that, if a patient was declared permanently unconscious, it was not unethical to discontinue all means of life-prolonging medical treatment (9) and this was reiterated in 1990 (10). In 1987, a judge in the Supreme Court of New Jersey declared that the convention that allowed withdrawal of life-sustaining treatment only from patients with a short expectation of life should not apply to a vegetative patient because it assumed that there was at least some benefit to be derived from continued sustenance (11). He went on to declare that, as vegetative patients could not experience any pain, suffering, joy, satisfaction or well-being, any analysis of benefits and burdens could not apply to them.

By 1990, there had been 26 court cases in 16 American states for withdrawal of life-sustaining treatment from vegetative patients (12). Then came the *Cruzan* case that led to extensive coverage in the American public media and medical literature as it made its way through several lower courts before the 1990 hearing in the US Supreme Court (p. 198). The final decision confirmed the appropriateness of withdrawing life-sustaining treatment, including ANH, from a vegetative patient, and most comment was supportive of this. Disagreements between the justices, as well as subsequent controversy, centred on who should make the decision to stop treatment rather than on the appropriateness of the decision. However, Justice William Brennan did note that it was improper to imply that 'continued existence and treatment in a persistent vegetative state is either beneficial or neutral. In fact not to terminate life-support robs a patient of the very qualities protected by the right to avoid unwanted medical treatment. A degraded existence is perpetuated; his family's suffering is protracted; and the memory he leaves behind becomes more and more distorted' (13).

Throughout most of this period, the UK remained silent on this topic, apart from the brief reference to vegetative children already mentioned (6). The British Medical Association's (BMA) report on euthanasia in 1988 commented that feeding tubes for nutrition and hydration were warranted only when 'they make possible a decent life in which the patient can reasonably be thought to have a continued interest' (14). It also asserted that a vegetative patient was in a state that could no longer be called a human life and thus it was futile to prolong it. However, this part of the report attracted little attention from commentators, who were more concerned with its strong stand against euthanasia (15). In 1991, a working party of the Institute of Medical Ethics in London considered it morally justified to withdraw ANH from PVS patients as 'it is difficult to see how prolonged survival in this non-sentient and undignified state can be in the best interests of the patient' (16). In 1992 a discussion paper from the BMA Medical Ethics Committee on the treatment of permanently vegetative patients confirmed its support for withdrawal of ANH, provided that two additional doctors had declared that the condition was permanent (17). This was relied on in the legal deliberations on the *Bland* case in 1992–93 in which nine judges in three successive English courts unanimously supported the withdrawal of ANH (18). These judges had various comments on the condition of the teenager *Bland* (p. 207). 'I cannot conceive what benefit his continued existence could be thought to give him', wrote one. 'The pitiful and humiliating helplessness of the vegetative patient offends the values of human dignity and personal privacy that belong to every person', said another. 'There is no question of *Bland*'s life being a life not worth living because the stark reality is that he has no life at all, and treatment serves no useful function', said a third, and another, 'Treatment can no longer serve to maintain the combination of manifold characteristics which we call a personality; he has no interests'.

In contrast to these detached medical and judicial views are the results of asking groups of people about their wishes for treatment if they were to become vegetative. In one study in 1989, 200 medical in-patients in Los Angeles were asked whether they would want life-support measures (intensive care, ventilation or dialysis) in various situations (19). Given a hopeless prognosis, 16% still wanted life support, but if they were to be left vegetative only 6% wanted such treatment. A more extensive study in Boston in 1988 involved 405 outpatients and 102 members of the public who were asked about what treatments they would refuse in an advance directive, given four different clinical scenarios leading to incompetence with a poor prognosis (20). If permanently vegetative or demented with terminal illness, over 80% would opt not to have any of five major life-saving or life-sustaining medical treatments offered (Table 6.2). Artificial nutrition was the least invasive of the treatments, yet it was refused as often as the other interventions.

Table 6.2. No treatment wishes (%) for four scenarios (*n* = 507)

Treatment refused	Dementia with terminal illness	PVS	Dementia	Coma – small chance of recovery
Cardiopulmonary rescue (CPR)	84	83	72	55
Major surgery	85	83	77	61
Ventilator	84	80	75	55
Dialysis	83	80	75	57
Artificial nutrition	82	80	76	60

From data in Emanuel et al. (20).

Table 6.3. No treatment wishes (%) for professionals themselves

	PVS	Dementia with terminal illness	Dementia	Coma – small chance of recovery
Physicians (*n* = 115)	90	89	75	51
Nurses (*n* = 127)	89	88	78	69

From Gillick et al. (21).

A later study in Boston using the same four scenarios involved physicians and nurses (21). Over two-thirds of the nurses were Catholic and almost half the physicians were Jewish, yet most of them would refuse treatment for themselves in several situations, especially if in a permanent VS (Table 6.3). When all four scenarios were combined, fewer would refuse nutrition (Table 6.4), presumably reflecting the lower refusal rate for nutrition in those in coma or with uncomplicated dementia shown in the previous study (Table 6.2). This report referred to an earlier survey of 345 private practice physicians in North Carolina, 93% of whom would refuse cardiopulmonary resuscitation (CPR) and 92% tube feeding if in permanent VS (22). A national survey of 169 neurologists and 150 nursing-home directors in the US found that 94% of both groups considered that a patient in permanent VS would be better off dead (23). This was in spite of some 12% believing that some vegetative patients had some awareness. The responses of the two groups to questions about the provision and withdrawal of life-saving or life-sustaining treatments were also similar, but in

Table 6.4. Refusal rate for various treatments (doctors + nurses, all scenarios)

Treatment	Refusal rate (% of 242)
Dialysis	88
CPR	86
Surgery	85
Ventilator	85
ANH	71

From Gillick et al. (21).

Table 6.5. Treatment preferences of physicians (%)

	Nursing-home directors ($n = 150$)			Neurologists ($n = 169$)		
Treatment	Usually provide	Would withdraw	Want for self	Usually provide	Would withdraw	Want for self
CPR	3	97	1	2	99	1
Ventilator	3	96	1	7	98	6
Dialysis	2	93	1	3	96	2
Antibiotic	34	93	8	31	96	6
ANH	29	89	10	47	88	13

From Payne et al. (23).

both groups fewer would want these treatments for themselves than would generally provide them for their patients (Table 6.5). A questionnaire to 114 American bioethics consultants found that only 10% wished to have nutrition continued if they were permanently vegetative (24). A complex study of health-state preferences in 40 well adults and 41 nursing-home residents in Seattle found that some considered dementia better than death but the majority rated coma (i.e. VS) as equal to or worse than death (25).

In a survey of 1027 UK doctors, 73% considered it sometimes appropriate to withdraw ANH from vegetative patients and, of these, over 90% would do so if the prognosis was permanent VS (26). Neurologists, neurosurgeons and orthopaedic surgeons made similar responses, but slightly fewer rehabilitationists would do so. When the same question was posed to doctors in six other European countries there were wide variations for ever withdrawing ANH (14–70%), the figure being less than a quarter for

Table 6.6. Japanese physicians (%) who would withdraw ANH (*n* = 190)

Patient's wish	Family's wish	Withdraw ANH (95% confidence)
Unknown	Unknown	3 (2–4)
Unknown	No LST	6 (4–8)
No LST	No LST	17 (36–44)

ANH, artificial nutrition and hydration; LST, life-sustaining treatment.
From Asai et al. (28).

France, Germany and Greece (27). In Mediterranean and Eastern European countries there is usually a presumption to continue to treat. Of those in the European study who would sometimes withdraw, 76–100% would consider this justified if the VS was permanent.

Very few of 190 members of the Japanese Apoplexy Society would withdraw ANH from a patient aged 70 years who had been vegetative for 2 years, even if the patient and family had requested this (Table 6.6); but 40% of these physicians would wish withdrawal of ANH for themselves in these circumstances (28). About half of these physicians considered that the dignity of the patient was only slightly or not at all offended by being in a vegetative state. Of these respondents, 30% had been requested at some time by family members to withdraw ANH, 73% to withhold dialysis or ventilation, and 77% to withhold CPR. This study noted that in a Japanese public opinion poll at least 25% did not want to be sustained if in permanent VS. A previous public poll had found that 80% would want treatment withdrawal for themselves but only 68% would ask for treatment to be withdrawn from a family member (29).

The Appleton International Conference on life-prolonging treatment in 1992 concluded that the permanently vegetative patient had no self-regarding interests and that there was no patient-based reason to continue life-sustaining treatment (30). There were, however, a number of dissenters from this view who believed that other moral interests might be at stake. It seems reasonable to assume that those who favour withholding or withdrawing life-prolonging treatment consider that the permanent vegetative state is equivalent to or worse than death. It does not follow that all those who do not support treatment withdrawal consider that survival in a vegetative state is of benefit to the patient or is an acceptable outcome of medical treatment. Some belong to the small minority who maintain that life in any state is an inherent good, but this vitalist position has been specifically rejected by many judges, religious leaders and philosophers, as it was by the Appleton Conference. It did not agree with the simple assumption that life itself was of paramount value irrespective of its quality and that, therefore, prolonging life was always in a patient's interest (30).

There are also those who warn about the wider implications of declaring or accepting that any person's life is not worth living. They challenge the right of anyone to make statements about the quality of life of another person, especially when these are made by a healthy individual. Some even doubt the validity of an advance directive, maintaining that the previously well patient who made it is different from the presently disabled person. For some, the concern seems less with the fate of an individual patient than with the supposed consequences of allowing permanently VS patients to be considered better off dead – the slippery slope argument. They fear that this might seem to legitimize euthanasia, and that in time such a judgement might be made about other severely disabled patients, in particular the demented and the elderly. In that context it is interesting that the American Geriatric Society submitted a brief as *amicus curiae* to the US Supreme Court in support of withdrawing ANH from *Nancy Cruzan*, fearing that elderly people would otherwise not be allowed to die when this was appropriate (31).

The belief that vegetative patients do not suffer is used as another argument for allowing them to survive indefinitely, and for asserting that allowing them to die is more for the benefit of the relatives than of the patient. Counter to this is the benefit that some families seem to gain from devoting time and energy to caring for the patient or from visiting regularly, but other commentators have expressed concern that maintaining life support for this reason could be regarded as sacrificing the interests of the patient to those of the relatives. Certainly, most seem to wish their vegetative relative to be kept alive. In the UK, where a court order is needed before ANH can be withdrawn, there have been only 25 such applications in the 7 years since the *Bland* judgement. The attitudes of the family members of 33 vegetative patients in American nursing homes have been studied (32). All had been vegetative for more than a year, some for more than 5 years; most were elderly, two-thirds of them over 70 years when they became vegetative. Most families wanted interventions for acute complications – antibiotics, transfer to an acute hospital and necessary surgery. However, 76% did not want their relative to have CPR or to be put on a ventilator although only 18% were in favour of discontinuing tube feeding. This contrasts strikingly with the 68% of people in a public survey in Japan who said that they would request withdrawal of ANH from a vegetative relative (29), although most doctors in that country would be unwilling to comply with such a request (28). People may respond differently to an imagined scenario than when confronted with an actual vegetative relative. The willingness of families to consider withholding new life-saving interventions, such as CPR, ventilation or antibiotics, even if they are uneasy about withdrawal of ANH, suggests that they would in fact welcome the death of their relative. They are not alone in claiming a special status for ANH among life-prolonging interventions, regardless of the interests of the patient (p. 108). Families vary in their reaction to PVS in a relative, and usually go through different phases as time passes until they accept that the condition is permanent (33). Some eventually reflect that it would have been better if the initial rescue and intensive care efforts had not been successful in saving their relative's life. The mother of one of my patients summed up the view of many relatives when she said, 'My son died at the roadside and the funeral was six years later'.

Some philosophers have maintained that permanently unconscious patients should be declared dead, on the grounds that they are no longer persons (34,35). They argue that this higher-brain definition of death is more logical than the whole-brain or brain-stem definitions of brain death. This view maintains that personhood depends on a biographical and relational life, not a merely biological one. However, the President's Commission rejected the proposal for this definition of death because it would be likely to create problems for social order (8). A suggested possible solution would be to build on the conscience clause in the New Jersey brain-death law that allows religious objectors to insist on cardiac stoppage rather than accepting whole-brain criteria (36). The argument is that personal choice on how your own death is declared should be allowed more widely than on religious grounds, and that the options should include the higher-brain definition. Another suggestion is that it might be more appropriate to invoke the fuzzy set of logicians and regard PVS patients as nonpersons who are not dead (37). There are certainly practical objections to a definition of death based on unconsciousness (38). One is the uncertainty of diagnosis and prognosis in our present state of knowledge. Another is that it might begin a slippery slope with a temptation to declare dead other patients with less devastating impairments of brain

function. Then there is the problem of contemplating the burial or crema-
tion of someone who is breathing and reflexly responsive. In practice there
would be a need to end biological life by a lethal injection or stopping
ANH. For these reasons, most physicians have been reluctant to adopt this
approach but in the survey of 319 American physicians almost half considered PVS patients to be already dead (23).

What of the minimally conscious state?

In contrast to the consensus about the vegetative state, there is much
controversy about the benefit to patients of regaining some evidence of
consciousness but remaining speechless, tube fed and totally dependent,
with only limited means of communication. Whilst any recovery may be
greeted as good, particularly by the family, there are those who question the
value of such a limited recovery. When the courts denied applications for
withdrawal of ANH from two minimally conscious American patients
(p. 142), medical comment was 'Being kept alive in a minimally conscious
state may be far worse than being maintained in a vegetative state. Precisely
because they are conscious they may suffer for years' (39). A British
television documentary called 'Waking from coma' showed two patients
with very limited recovery but better than minimally conscious. The
response of several broadsheet TV critics was that these patients would
have been better off if they had been still vegetative or had died. Many years
ago, a substantial minority voted recovery to very severe disability as being
worse than remaining vegetative, which was regarded as worse than death
(Table 6.1) (4).

Those who express such views are healthy people, many without direct
experience of severely disabled patients. Rehabilitationists who are familiar
with the capacity of patients to adapt to major disability that they would
previously have considered unacceptable tend to think otherwise. However, it is doubtful how valid it is to extrapolate from patients whose brains
are intact but have severe physical disability to those with profound brain
damage. In reporting the limited recovery of 11 previously vegetative
patients, Andrews (40) commented that most patients showed no evidence
of depression or of feeling that their condition was worse than nonsenti-
ence or death. He admitted that this was a subjective impression based on
observing signs of pleasure more often than of distress. He added that

Table 6.7. Decisions to limit treatment for different predicted outcomes

Predicted outcome	Withhold acute interventions ($n = 1594$) %	Withdraw ANH ($n = 1152$) %
Vegetative	92	92
Minimally conscious	31	22
Very severely disabled	14	12

Minimally conscious = no speech, able to communicate simple needs. Very severely disabled = able to speak, totally dependent, insight re condition. Applies to patients still in VS; n = number of doctors who consider such treatment limitation sometimes appropriate.
From data in survey of European doctors (27).

distress was more common in those who had good insight, implying that some were too cognitively impaired to appreciate their plight.

It is possible to underestimate the degree of awareness and capacity for cognitive function in these patients. Skilled personnel using a buzzer for yes/no responses to questions, or a pointer and letter board to allow freer expression, may discover much more responsiveness than an average observer would expect. One case where expert neurologists found very little reliable responsiveness was investigated by two different specially-trained psychologists in two sessions of two days each. Responses by pressing a buzzer revealed in the patient considerable autobiographical memory, and the ability to learn some verbal tasks and to express a view that she wanted life-sustaining treatment to be continued (41,42). This provoked a thoughtful review of the validity of decision making by patients in a minimally conscious state that suggested that limited consciousness can give potential for some positive as well as negative experiences (43).

To find out what doctors think about these outcomes, the European study enquired about withdrawing life-prolonging treatment from vegetative patients according to the predicted final outcome (Table 6.7). If predicted to be in what we would now call a minimally conscious state, a third of British doctors and more than a fifth of doctors in five other countries would withhold treatment for life-threatening conditions from a vegetative patient (range 15–39%). For withdrawing ANH the range was 13–29%. For patients predicted to remain with very severe disability but better than minimally conscious, if any recovery did occur a small minority of doctors would also limit treatment for patients who were still vegetative. Clearly, some doctors are prepared to act on the assumption that the minimally conscious state or even very severe disability is no better than the vegetative state.

It is clear that the majority of those questioned support the withdrawal of life-prolonging treatment from permanently vegetative patients, and indeed this has been sanctioned by many institutional statements and supported by many courts of law, as well as by most comment in the media. Certainly most people in several countries appear to consider that indefinite survival in the vegetative state is worse than death.

REFERENCES

1 Thompson GT. An appeal to doctors. *Lancet* 1969; 2: 1353

2 *Lancet.* Death of a human being. *Lancet* 1971; 2: 590–91

3 Bishop of Durham. Moral problems facing the medical problem at the present time. *The Bishoprick* 1972; 47: 48–61

4 Jennett B. Resource allocation for the severely brain damaged. *Arch Neurol* 1976; 33: 595–7

5 Feinberg WM, Ferry PC. A fate worse than death: the persistent vegetative state in childhood. *Am J Disab Child* 1984; 138: 128–30

6 Campbell AGM. Children in a persistent vegetative state. *BMJ* 1984; 289: 1022–3

7 Timmins N. A fate worse than death. *The Independent* (London newspaper) 1987; 30th March

8 President's Commission for the study of Ethical Problems in Medicine. *Deciding to forego life-sustaining treatment.* Washington DC: US Government Printing Office, 1983

9 American Medical Association Council on Ethical and Judicial Affairs. Statement on withholding or withdrawing life-prolonging medical treatment. *JAMA* 1986; 256: 471

10 American Medical Association Councils on Scientific Affairs and on Ethical and Judicial Affairs. Persistent vegetative state and the decision to withdraw or withhold life support. *JAMA* 1990; 263: 426–30

11 *In re Peter* 108 NJ 365, 529 A2d 419 (1987)

12 Weir RF, Gostin L. Decisions to abate life-sustaining treatment for nonautonomous patients. *JAMA* 1990; 264: 1846–53

13 *Cruzan* v. *Director,* Missouri Dept of Health 110 S. Ct. 2841 (1990)

14 Working party of the British Medical Association. *The euthanasia report.* London: BMA, 1988

15 Higgs R. Not the last word on euthanasia. *BMJ* 1988; 296: 1348

16 Institute of Medical Ethics Working Party. Withdrawal of life-support from patients in a persistent vegetative state. *Lancet* 1991; 337: 96–8

17 Medical Ethics Committee of the British Medical Association. *Discussion paper on treatment of patients in persistent vegetative state.* London: BMA, 1992

18 *Airedale NHS Trust* v. *Bland* [1993] 1 All ER 821

19 Frankl D, Oye RK, Bellamy PE. Attitudes of hospitalized patients towards life support: a survey of 200 medical inpatients. *Amer J Med* 1989; 86: 645–8

20 Emanuel LL, Barry MJ, Stoeckle JD et al. Advance directives for medical care – a case for greater use. *N Engl J Med* 1991; 324: 889–95

21 Gillick MR, Hesse K, Mazzapica N. Medical technology at the end of life: what would physicians and nurses want for themselves? *Arch Intern Med* 1993; 153: 2542–7

22 Brunetti L, Carperos S, Westlund R. Physicians' attitudes towards living wills and cardiopulmonary resuscitation. *J Gen Intern Med* 1991; 6: 323–9

23 Payne K, Taylor RM, Stocking C et al. Physicians' attitudes about the care of patients in the persistent vegetative state: a national survey. *Ann Intern Med* 1996; 125: 104–10

24 Fox E, Stocking C. Ethics consultants' recommendations for life-prolonging treatment of patients in a persistent vegetative state. *JAMA* 1993; 270: 2578–82

25 Patrick DL, Starks HE, Cain KC et al. Measuring preferences for health states worse than death. *Med Decis Making* 1994; 14: 9–18

26 Grubb A, Walsh P, Lambe N et al. Survey of British clinicians' views on management of patients in persistent vegetative state. *Lancet* 1996; 348: 35–40

27 Grubb A, Walsh P, Lambe N et al. *The moral and legal issues surrounding the treatment and care of patients in persistent vegetative state.* Report to European Biomedical and Health Research Programme. 1997 [on file in the library of the Centre of Medical Law and Ethics, King's College, London]

28 Asai A, Maekawa M, Akiguchi I et al. Survey of Japanese physicians' attitudes towards the care of adult patients in persistent vegetative state. *J Med Ethics* 1999; 25: 302–8

29 Winslade WJ. *Permanently unconscious patients: the need for responsible medical, legal, and public policies.* Unpublished report of international conference in Bellagio, Italy. 1994

30 Stanley JM. The Appleton International Conference: developing guidelines for decisions to forgo life-prolonging medical treatment. *J Med Ethics* 1992; 18: 3–22

31 Glover JJ. The case of Ms Cruzan and the care of the elderly. *J Am Geriatr Soc* 1990; 38: 588–93

32 Tresch DD, Sims FH, Duthie EH et al. Patients in a persistent vegetative state: attitudes and reactions of family members. *J Am Geriatr Soc* 1991; 39: 17–21

33 Jacobs HE, Muir CA, Cline JD. Family reactions to persistent vegetative state. *J Head*

Trauma Rehabil 1986; 1: 55–62

34 Veatch RM. The whole-brain-oriented concept of death: an outmoded philosophical foundation. *J Thanatol* 1975; 3: 13–30

35 Gervais KG. *Redfining death.* New Haven, Yale University Press, 1997

36 Veatch RM. The conscience clause. In *The Definition of Death.* Youngner SJ, Arnold
RM, Schapiro R. (Eds). Baltimore: Johns Hopkins University Press, 1999: 137–60

37 Brody B. Special ethical issues in the management of PVS patients. *Law Med Health
Care* 1992; 20: 104–15

38 Schrode KE. Life in limbo: revising policies for permanently unconscious patients.
Houston Law Rev 1995; 31: 1610–67

39 Nelson LJ, Cranford RE. Michael Martin and Robert Wendland: beyond the
vegetative state. *J Contemp Health Law Policy* 1999; 15: 427–53

40 Andrews K. Recovery of patients after four months or more in the persistent
vegetative state. *BMJ* 1993; 306: 1597–1600

41 McMillan TM. Neuropsychological assessment after extremely severe head injury in
a case of life or death. *Brain Injury* 1997; 11: 483–90

42 Shiel A, Wilson BA. Assessment after extremely severe head injury in a case of life or
death: further support for McMillan. *Brain Injury* 1998; 12: 809–16

43 Phipps E, Whyte J. Medical decision-making with persons who are minimally
conscious: a commentary. *Am J Phys Med Rehabil* 1999; 78: 77–82

7

Medical management

This chapter briefly reviews the principles of medical treatment for patients in the vegetative state but without discussing the details of techniques that depend on the expertise of therapists in rehabilitation teams. The significance of the setting in which these patients are treated is important to recognize. Because this condition is relatively rare, any one hospital or doctor is unlikely to encounter more than the occasional vegetative patient, with the exception of the very few rehabilitation units that have a special interest in this condition. In a review of over 1000 UK doctors in specialities likely to encounter vegetative patients 46% had never encountered one, 31% had seen less than five and only 10% more than ten (1).

In the early stages these patients are in acute units – neurosurgical, orthopaedic, neurological, medical or intensive care. In many places there is pressure to discharge these patients early from such acute settings, but there are very few rehabilitation units willing or able to take such dependent patients within a few weeks of the acute insult. There are some units of this kind in the USA but for patients that reach them there are often difficulties in maintaining funding for more than a month or so of treatment unless the patient is already showing enough improvement to claim that active rehabilitation should continue to be supported. As a result many of these patients are soon transferred to nursing homes with skilled nursing facilities but which do not have specialized rehabilitation programmes.

In the UK, by contrast, these patients often remain for many weeks and sometimes months in acute medical or surgical units where, again, there are no special skills in the rehabilitation of severely brain-damaged patients. Most rehabilitation units are reluctant to take a nonresponsive patient who is considered unlikely to be able to participate in an active programme. Where there are units that specialize in the management of severely disabled survivors after brain damage, most reports reveal that many of their patients come as secondary referrals, often many months after their acute illness, usually as a result of pressure from the family. By this time, many patients are already suffering from complications such as contractures and malnutrition. Given the patchy pattern of early care, it is not surprising that some rehabilitationists believe that some vegetative patients fail to reach their full potential for recovery. Most patients, including those who reach a special unit but who remain vegetative, will eventually be transferred for long-term care to a chronic-care hospital unit, a nursing home or charitable institution or, with suitable support, to their family home. It is against this background that the recommendations from groups of experts that are summarized below have to be read.

The aim of early management is to provide the best conditions for recovery to occur and to ensure that those who do make some recovery are able, when the time comes, to make the most of any returning neurological function. Measures are directed towards maintaining the patient in the best possible general condition, by ensuring good skin care and nutrition, and minimizing muscle contractures (2,3,4,5). Patients a few weeks after their brain damage will usually have a nasogastric tube for nutrition and hydration. This may cause local irritation and is liable to cause aspiration of gastric contents into the respiratory tract by regurgitation through an oesophageal sphincter rendered incompetent by the tube. Once it is clear that the patient is remaining vegetative, it is best to establish a percutaneous endoscopic gastrostomy (PEG) (6). This entails inserting a wide-bore tube directly into the stomach through the skin and it avoids any irritation to the nose or the oesophagus. It is then possible to undertake most feeding by continuous drip through the night when the patient is immobile, thus minimizing any postural regurgitation when the patient is moved by nurses and therapists during the day. Several weeks or months after the acute episode many transferred patients are found to be underweight, with a low body mass index. To bring them up to their ideal body weight dieticians should determine the appropriate intake, adjusted as necessary if there is diarrhoea. Good nutrition makes it easier to maintain an intact skin and for the patient to resist infective complications. Once up to their normal weight, it is equally important to guard against obesity as this can make nursing more difficult, as well as posing a problem for those patients who get to the stage of regaining some mobility.

Chest complications can be a threat to life, and care is needed to avoid aspiration either of gastric contents or of saliva by providing regular suction when necessary. Oral and dental hygiene need regular attention. If there is a tracheostomy it should be closed as soon as possible. In the event of respiratory infection, chest physiotherapy and antibiotics are needed. Good skin condition and avoidance of decubitus ulcers depends on regular skin care and frequent changes of position. Special mattresses designed to alternate areas of pressure are useful. An in-dwelling bladder catheter predisposes to infection and condom drainage is a better alternative in males. Bowel evacuation can usually be adequately dealt with by regular suppositories but enemas may sometimes be needed.

Regular passive movements of the limb joints through their normal range of motion are essential. If increased tone becomes a major problem there may be a case for antispastic drugs, occasionally for nerve blocks. Sessions sitting out of bed can be of benefit in relaxing spasm and some think that they promote arousal. Special seating is needed, with support for the head that cannot usually be held up (7). Some physiotherapists like their patients to graduate to standing sessions strapped to a tilting table, but the benefits of this are dubious.

No one would question the appropriateness of the supportive measures outlined above, although in practice there are wide variations in the vigour with which some are applied, and for how long. More contentious is the value of certain other treatments that some have claimed might promote emergence from the vegetative state. The Task Force began its section on treatment with the assertion that no such therapies had been reliably shown to be successful. The problem is the difficulty of establishing the efficacy of interventions when the number of patients is so small that formal trials are not practical. Most reports are observations on single patients whom it is believed were better after a given intervention. Some improvement in arousal or responsiveness is often the basis of such a belief. Not only may these represent the natural evolution of the condition but they may not be associated with any overall benefit to the patient. Sometimes the claim is made that an intervention was followed by improvement only weeks or months later. As it is so difficult to predict which individual vegetative patients will show any recovery, and when that is likely to occur, it is usually impossible to rule out spontaneous recovery as the explanation for improvement attributed by its advocates to a given intervention. It is worth noting that none of the reports of unexpected late recoveries have claimed that these followed a recent change of treatment that might have accounted for the return of consciousness.

Sensory stimulation, sometimes termed a 'coma arousal programme', is the treatment that has most often been claimed to promote arousal and behavioural responsiveness. One theoretical basis for such a programme is that it reduces sensory deprivation, which is known to have harmful effects on behaviour in normal persons. It is certainly likely that vegetative patients do suffer a degree of sensory deprivation by reason of their brain damage. Another rationale is that because the developing brain in the young child responds well to increased sensory experience it is supposed that the brain that is recovering from severe damage might react similarly. Families and professional carers normally indulge in conversation with the unresponsive patient, play music and display family and other photographs – in the hope that these may capture the attention of the patient as soon as there is any return of consciousness and might therefore promote further recovery. The question is whether a systematic programme of sensory input, aimed specifically at certain senses and repeated at regular intervals, is any more effective than the informal stimulation provided by carers and families. An extensive review in 1996 concluded that there was very little adequate research indicating the effectiveness of such programmes (8).

Pharmacological interventions, such as the use of dopamine agonists or dextroamphetamines, have been tried sporadically but with no convincing evidence of effectiveness (9). All are agreed, however, about the importance of reviewing the drugs being given for other purposes (e.g. antispastics and anticonvulsants) lest their sedative effects are impairing the detection of returning responsiveness. It is more than 10 years since a number of reports from Japan of the benefits of electrical stimulation of the mesencephalic reticular formation or the thalamic nuclei in promoting arousal (10), but the evidence for benefit was not clear and this approach has not been taken up elsewhere.

As the weeks and months pass, so the treatment of vegetative patients changes in its aims and emphasis. In the early weeks there will usually be full technological support as required – intensive care, ventilation, surgical interventions and drug treatment for complications, and even dialysis and cardiopulmonary resuscitation (CPR) if the need arises. After some months, if there are no signs of improvement, active rehabilitation may be scaled down, often at the request of relatives who consider that their relative is more bothered than helped by continuing efforts, for example, to sit him out of bed for long periods. It may be agreed with the family not to embark on new technological interventions in the event of complications. This reflects the widespread view that indefinite survival in a vegetative or even a very severely disabled state is worse than death, as reviewed in Chapter 6. None the less many families with a vegetative relative do ask for all active medical treatment to be continued, including dealing with new complications, even when no recovery is expected (pp. 80, 81). This may reflect a lingering hope that a miraculous recovery may still occur, or the need for more time to come to terms with the permanence of the patient's condition.

Most families do eventually agree to a do not resuscitate (DNR) order and that there should not be any other new acute technological interventions for complications, and some agree also that antibiotics should not be given for any infections that occur. Such decisions are commonly made much sooner than the vegetative state can be declared permanent by the criteria of the US Task Force. They are presumably made on the same basis as they commonly are about many other seriously ill patients with a low probability of a reasonable or acceptable recovery. The evidence for this comes partly from personal experience and from informal reports from colleagues, but there are also systematic data from a survey of doctors' attitudes in seven European countries (11). In five countries, 78–100% of doctors considered it sometimes appropriate to withhold treatment for infections or other life-threatening conditions. The doctors who were prepared to withhold these treatments were then asked how soon it was appropriate to consider such a decision. Overall, 16% would do so in the first 3 months (range 8–33% between countries), and 31% would do so between 4 and 6 months (range 13–35%). These figures reflect the number of doctors who were very or quite confident of predicting the ultimate outcome at each of these time periods – 17% and 38% respectively. The questionnaire to these doctors referred briefly to the Task Force report for the definition of the vegetative state, but it is not known how widely its conclusions on prognosis were known among the European doctors when their views were surveyed.

Once the vegetative state is declared permanent the phase of palliative care is reached, when ANH and full nursing care is continued but there is no longer an active programme of rehabilitation. By this stage, there is almost always a DNR order and usually an agreement about no new interventions or antibiotics. In the event of a patient already on dialysis who had then suffered a hypoxic incident leading to a permanent VS it would be appropriate at this stage to discontinue dialysis – and a protocol for doing so has been published (12). Sometimes, even at this stage, a family may insist on full technological treatment for complications and refuse to agree even to a DNR order (13). They may not give reasons other than that this is their wish, but some claim that religious beliefs oblige them to request that life be preserved by all means possible. The reactions of hospitals and courts to demands for futile treatment are discussed later (p. 140).

The question of withdrawing ANH may now be considered by the family and the treating team because of the evidence that even with a decision to withhold new interventions patients who have survived this long may live for many years. However, a decision to withdraw is actually taken in only a small minority of cases. Although some 80–90% of those questioned wished ANH to be discontinued if they themselves were vegetative (see Tables 6.2–6.5), only 57% of the doctors in the European survey were willing to consider withdrawal from their patients in a permanent VS (range 14–73% between countries). This is fewer than would consider withholding acute interventions for new complications (79%). However, of those who would withdraw ANH the proportion who would do so in the first 3 months (12%), or between 4 and 6 months (24%), was not much lower than would withhold new interventions (16% and 31%). In a study of the attitudes of American physicians (14), very similar results were obtained about their willingness to limit life-prolonging treatment (see Table 6.5). Questioned a year before the Task Force data on prognosis, these American physicians replied that the vegetative state could be considered permanent at 4–8 weeks after hypoxic brain damage and at 8–10 weeks after head injury.

The European doctors were asked about what factors would influence their decisions to limit life-prolonging treatment. The most important factor was naturally their estimate of the ultimate outcome. However, some doctors were prepared to limit treatment even when the patient was predicted to make some partial recovery from the vegetative state (see Table 6.7). This probably explains the willingness of some doctors to limit treatment before they are confident that the patient will remain permanently vegetative. Asked to rank various factors as the most important in influencing their decision, the front runner was how long the patient had been vegetative; 48% ranked this first for withholding interventions and 54% for withdrawing ANH. The age of the patient ranked first for 20% in withholding decisions and 17% in withdrawing. The cause of injury, an important prognostic factor in the Task Force report, ranked first for only 10% of doctors deciding to withhold and for 8% before withdrawing ANH.

The withdrawal of ANH raises ethical and legal issues more often than does the withholding of life-saving treatments for new complications. These issues are dealt with at length later (pp. 108–13). They mainly centre on the debate about whether ANH is medical treatment that, if not beneficial, can be withdrawn, or whether it is regarded as part of basic nursing care to which every patient has a continuing right. Physicians and nurses should be reassured by the many position statements from professional bodies on both sides of the Atlantic approving the withdrawal of ANH from permanently vegetative patients. There are also numerous court judgements affirming the legality of such a management decision in appropriate circumstances. The concern here is not with these controversies but with the practicalities of withdrawing ANH.

Perhaps the main reluctance to take this decision is the fear that there will be unpleasant consequences for the patient and the onlookers, such as those associated with starvation and hydration in people shipwrecked or lost in the desert. A strikingly titled paper 'The sloganism of starvation' reported how lawyers in several American courts who were opposed to withdrawal had painted pictures of a cruel, painful and gruesome death if ANH was withdrawn (15). It went on to quote several reports of terminal dehydration in dying patients who were still conscious that indicated that this usually resulted in depression of consciousness and no obvious distress. Since then there have been many reports of a peaceful death, free of distress for the carers, following the withdrawal of food and fluid in terminally ill patients (16,17,18). Most of these reports were about elderly patients and the support of the American Geriatrics Society for the withdrawal of ANH from *Nancy Cruzan* in its *amicus curiae* to the US Supreme Court has been noted (pp. 80, 111). Moreover, the American Academy of Neurology has recommended that profoundly and irreversibly paralysed patients with retained consciousness and cognition should be allowed to die by refusing nutrition and hydration (19,20). The consensus is that soon after withdrawal there is a release of opioids with an analgesic effect; later hypernatraemia and ketonaemia give rise to confusion and eventually coma in these initially conscious patients (21). Whilst it can be argued that vegetative patients cannot suffer, these data are reassuring for those who do believe that some residual awareness may remain in some vegetative patients. Renal failure is probably the final cause of death, but hypovolaemia may lead to reduced cardiac output and cerebral blood flow. Death normally occurs peacefully in 8–14 days.

The other concern is that withdrawing the symbolic act of offering food and fluid to a patient indicates that he is being abandoned. It is important therefore to emphasize to the family and professional carers that all other nursing care will continue. The patient will be turned, have regular skin care and the dry mouth that occurs will be dealt with by oral hygiene and moistening the lips with ice-chips and wet swabs (21). A nursing paper on this topic captured the situation in its title 'We withdrew nutrition – not care' (22). Nurses involved should be given every opportunity to discuss the implications of a decision to withdraw ANH, and to be offered support and counselling. There may, none the less, be some nurses who are unwilling to participate in the care of a patient during the withdrawal of ANH, and their concerns should be met by transfer to other duties.

In spite of many courts in the US declaring that withdrawal of ANH is legally acceptable without court review, many institutions in that country remain reluctant to allow it on their premises, perhaps for fear of bad publicity from pro-life activists. This is particularly so for nursing homes because of antiabuse regulations that are often mistakenly interpreted as mandating continued nutritional support (p. 141). The matter may be taken to court for an order to withdraw treatment but is more often dealt with by allowing the family to take the patient home with the support of the family physician. In the UK, where all cases have to go to court, most withdrawals are done in hospital but sometimes a family requests that the patient spends his last days at home and there is no problem about this if the general practitioner is supportive.

REFERENCES

1 Grubb A, Walsh P, Lambe N et al. Survey of British clinicians' views on management of persistent vegetative state. *Lancet* 1996; 348: 35–40

2 Andrews K. Managing the persistent vegetative state: early skilled treatment offers the best hope for optimal recovery. *BMJ* 1992; 305: 486–7

3 Andrews K. Patients in the persistent vegetative state: problems in their long term management. *BMJ* 1993; 306: 1600–602

4 Sandel ME. Medical management of the comatose, vegetative or minimally conscious patient. *Neurorehabilitation* 1996; 6: 9–17

5 Whyte J, Glenn MB. The care and rehabilitation of the patient in a persistent vegetative state. *J Head Trauma Rehabil* 1986; 1: 39–53

6 Park RHR, Allison MC, Lang J et al. Randomised comparison of percutaneous endoscopic gastrostomy and nasogastric tube feeding in patients with persisting neurological dysphagia. *BMJ* 1992; 304: 1406–9

7 Shaw R. Persistent vegetative state: principles and techniques for seating and positioning. *J Head Trauma Rehabil.* 1986; 1: 31–7

8 Giacino JT. Sensory stimulation: theoretical perspectives and the evidence for effectiveness. *Neurorehabilitation* 1996; 6: 69–78

9 Elovic E. Pharmacology of attention and arousal in the low level patient. *Neurorehabilitation* 1986; 6: 57–67

10 Tsubokawa T, Yamamoto T, Katayama Y et al. Deep-brain stimulation in a persistent vegetative state: follow-up results and criteria for selection of candidates. *Brain Inj* 1990; 4: 315–27

11 Grubb A, Walsh P, Lambe N et al. *The moral and legal issues surrounding the treatment and care of patients in persistent vegetative state.* Report to European Biomedical and Health Research Programme. 1997 [on file in the library of the Centre of Medical Law and Ethics, King's College, London]

12 Eiser AR, Seiden DJ. Discontinuing dialysis in persistent vegetative state: the roles of autonomy, community and professional moral agency. *Am J Kidney Dis* 1997; 30: 291–6

13 Weijer C. Cardiopulmonary resuscitation for patients in a persistent vegetative state: futile or acceptable? *CMAJ* 1998; 158: 491–3

14 Payne K, Taylor RM, Stocking C et al. Physicians' attitudes about the care of patients in the persistent vegetative state: a national survey. *Ann Intern Med* 1996; 125: 104–10

15 Ahronheim J, Gasner MR. The sloganism of starvation. *Lancet* 1990; 1: 278–9

16 Printz LA. Terminal dehydration, a compassionate treatment. *Arch Intern Med* 1992; 152: 697–700

17 Sullivan RJ. Accepting death without artificial nutrition or hydration. *J Gen Intern Med* 1993; 8: 220–24

18 Bernat JL, Gert B, Mogielnicki RP. Patient refusal of hydration and nutrition: an alternative to physician-assisted suicide or voluntary active euthanasia. *Arch Intern Med* 1993; 153: 2723–8

19 American Academy of Neurology. Position statement: certain aspects of the care and management of profoundly and irreversibly paralyzed patients with retained consciousness and cognition. *Neurology* 1993; 43: 222–3

20 Bernat JL, Cranford RE, Kittredge FI et al. Competent patients with advanced states

of permanent paralysis have the right to forgo life-sustaining therapy. *Neurology* 1993; 43: 224–5

21 Brody H, Campbell ML, Faber-Langendoen K et al. Withdrawing intensive life-sustaining treatment – recommendations for compassionate clinical management. *N Engl J Med* 1997; 336: 652–7

22 Ohlenberg E. We withdrew nutrition – not care. *RN* 1996; 59: 36–40

8

Ethical issues

It might seem impractical to attempt to separate discussion of the ethical and legal issues raised by decisions to limit life-prolonging treatment for vegetative patients, in that the law in these cases is largely concerned with the application of ethical principles to particular situations. Moreover, it is the courts that provide an opportunity for doctors and ethicists to seek the formal approval of the public or society, as represented by the judiciary, for what they see as appropriate decisions to limit treatment. More strictly legal issues are the development of procedures for making such a decision, in particular defining who should be consulted and whose views should be determinative in reaching a decision and what role the courts should play. It is these matters that will be dealt with in the remaining chapters. However, in discussing ethics there will inevitably be reference to some court cases because certain legal decisions have been crucial in the evolution and acceptance of some of the ethical attitudes that have come to inform contemporary medical practice. Moreover, high profile court cases have been important not just for establishing legal precedents or confirming previous judgements, but in the discussions they have provoked among physicians, ethicists and the public about the issues involved. There is therefore inevitably some overlap and repetition in the chapters dealing with ethical and legal issues.

It might be thought that the ethical principles would have been developed first, then the implications for the law of applying these would have been considered, and that only after that would physicians have deemed it safe to put them into practice. In fact, this has not been the sequence of events. Physicians began to make treatment-limiting decisions on the paternalistic basis of judging these to be in the best interests of their patients. Only later did some cases come for judicial review before treatment was limited, because either physicians or hospital attorneys were reluctant to proceed for fear of ensuing litigation. Ethicists appeared on the scene largely in response to publicized legal decisions, analysing the actions of physicians and lawyers and proposing principles that they maintained should inform future decision making. In deferring formal discussion of ethics until after describing public and professional opinions about the value of vegetative survival (see Chapter 6), and the practical implications of this for medical treatment (see Chapter 7) this book echoes this sequence.

This account begins with developments in the USA, where lawyers and ethicists have been engaging doctors in debate on this issue for many years. For some time before there was any detailed debate about vegetative patients, concern had been growing that some technologies designed to save lives, such as resuscitation and intensive care, appeared in some patients to do no more than to extend the dying process. In such circumstances physicians felt that the application of some life-prolonging treatments was doing more harm than good to patients. In 1957, a group of anaesthesiologists sought advice from Pope Pius XII who ruled that there was no obligation to use extraordinary means to prolong life in hopelessly ill patients (1). Ten years later came the definition of brain death by the Harvard criteria, with the implication that once this was diagnosed the ventilator could be withdrawn although the heart was still beating (2). Laws in several states subsequently accepted that death could be declared by neurological criteria. By the mid 1970s, clinicians began publishing about the need to withhold or withdraw life-prolonging treatments that were considered of no benefit to the patient, and the phrase 'death with dignity' emerged, particularly in intensive care settings (3).

It was against this background that the Supreme Court of New Jersey decided a landmark case in 1976 (4). *Karen Quinlan,* aged 21 was in a vegetative state following a cardiac arrest complicating drug-induced coma 9 months previously. Unusually, she was still on a ventilator and the court granted her father's request that he become her legal guardian and that he could then authorize the removal of the respirator and other supportive treatment to let her die (p. 189). The judge in this case acknowledged the legitimate roles of theology, medicine and the law in decisions of this kind. The Quinlans were devout Roman Catholics and the Catholic bishops of New Jersey submitted an *amicus curiae* affirming that discontinuing this extraordinary treatment would be morally correct, quoting the 1957 statement of the Pope. At that time, the only authoritative statement by a major medical organization formally approving limitation of treatment for patients who were not brain dead was that from the AMA in 1974 about do not resuscitate orders (5).

Principles of medical ethics

The 1970s saw the development of medical ethics as a major interest in the US, not only for physicians, but also for theologians and secular moral philosophers. Many academic appointments were made and independent bodies such as the Kennedy Institute and the Hastings Center were established, while many hospitals appointed bioethics consultants and set up Ethics Committees. The latter were to advise on protocols for dealing with difficult scenarios that occurred frequently and were therefore predictable as well as being available for consultation about decision making about individual patients when differing opinions had to be resolved. Medical ethics thus moved rapidly from a scholarly discipline of theoretical arguments to an essentially practical activity. Beauchamp and Childress in 1979 published a systematic analysis of the moral principles that should underline decision making in medicine (6). Their four basic principles of autonomy, beneficence, nonmaleficence and justice have stood the test of time, albeit that ethicists often differ in how to order the priorities when there is a conflict between these four (7). That there is often a need to balance competing principles is the essence of medical ethics, to the disappointment of some physicians who had hoped that their application in difficult situations would usually make the right decision obvious.

The most striking development of the ethics movement in the USA was the emergence of patient **autonomy** as the dominant ethical principle in medical practice. This was seen as replacing the paternalism of physicians, who had previously regarded it as their duty to decide what was best for the patient, in the expectation that their advice would be accepted. Indeed, Beauchamp later pointed out (8) that the British physician Thomas Percival who, in 1803, had written the first English-speaking doctrine of health-care ethics, had perceived this as a duty. Percival had stated that the doctor's view of what we now call beneficence and maleficence clearly took precedence over truthfully informing patients of the options for treatment, let alone allowing them to make their own decisions. These views dominated British and American practice for many years, being largely reproduced in the AMA's first code of ethics in 1847. It was later that autonomy, defined as deliberated self-rule, became recognized as important. This was most eloquently and forcibly expressed in John Stuart Mill's *On Liberty* in 1859 (9), which has been described as the classic text on antipaternalism. He wrote 'The only purpose for which power can be rightfully exercised over any member of a civilised community, against his will, is to prevent harm to others. His own good, either physical or moral, is not a sufficient warrant.'

In the context of medical treatment the patient can exercise autonomy only if truthfully informed by the physician of the pros and cons of all available alternatives. The expectation now is that the patient will make the decision about what is to be done, in partnership with the physician. Implicit in autonomy is that the patient may choose to hand back decision-making authority to the physician, or at least to invite him to become the dominant member of the partnership. Although frequently hailed as a recent development, the principle of patient autonomy was established legally in 1914 (10) and is embodied in the legal principle of consent (p. 129). It is therefore accepted in medical practice, although the persistence of paternalism among physicians has meant that until recently often only lip service was paid to it.

The dominance of autonomy over beneficence means that a patient may refuse treatment from which, in the view of others, the patient could derive some benefit, and that a request may be made for treatment already started to be discontinued, including life-prolonging treatment. Although normally such a refusal will be negotiated between the patient and the doctor, the President's Commission on forgoing life-sustaining treatment in 1983 emphasized that the decision must be based firmly on the values and goals of the patient rather than those of the doctor (11). It is assumed that a patient refusing treatment has decided that this particular intervention involves more burdens than benefits, but there is, in fact, no need for a patient to provide detailed justification for refusing treatment. Even if such a choice is considered unwise, a doctor must comply with the patient's wishes, provided that the patient is both competent and has been adequately informed of the likely consequences of refusal.

The pre-eminence of autonomy in American ethics may reflect a society founded on populations seeking freedom from oppressive regimes, and it has not been accepted as enthusiastically in some European countries or in Japan, where medical paternalism lingers. Some theologians also have questioned the wisdom of according autonomy such an overarching place in ethics, because it seems to enshrine selfishness as a good. They assert that the essence of human personhood lies in relationships with others. This may be countered by emphasizing that the autonomy principle requires that in exercising autonomy the patient should always respect the autonomy of others who may be affected by his decisions, such as family and carers. The main challenge to autonomy as justifying a right to refuse life-prolonging treatment comes from certain religious minorities that maintain that no man should make a decision that will hasten his death, as it is God who should determine when an individual life ends. Most orthodox Jews, together with some fundamentalist Protestants and conservative Roman Catholics, hold this version of the vitalist view. Finally, it should be noted that autonomy is not taken to extend to the right to demand treatment that has been deemed futile by the physician, but views differ about how to deal with such a request (pp. 106, 140). Nor does autonomy allow a patient to demand an illegal act, such as active euthanasia – although advocates of this practice have defined it as the ultimate autonomy.

With such strong support for the right of the competent patient to refuse treatment, there is a natural concern to find means of protecting the incompetent patient from treatment that would likely be refused if that were possible. Such a patient's autonomy can be truly exercised only if it is possible to discover what that patient would likely want in the present circumstance, and the American courts have identified means of ascertaining this (p. 130).

Beneficence could be considered to cover the basic goals of medicine. These are to restore function and health, to halt or slow the progress of disease, and to relieve symptoms and suffering. These could be summarized as to improve the quality of life of the patient. Prolonging life is not a basic goal because it is not necessarily always a benefit. Indeed all the delegates to the Appleton Conference rejected the vitalist assumption that life itself is of paramount value irrespective of quality, and that prolonging life is therefore always in a patient's best interest (12). Many people consider that prolonging life brings no benefit to a permanently vegetative patient (see Chapter 6).

Maleficence includes the risk, discomfort and indignity associated with treatment, as well as any added disability that results from treatment. It would also apply to prolonging suffering by continuing to treat. Serious burdens for the patient's family as a result of continuing treatment can also be counted as harmful. However, keeping a vegetative patient alive mainly for the supposed emotional benefits of the family or carers rather than for the patient's own benefit could be considered maleficence from the patient's perspective.

It is, of course, the balance between benefits and burdens that has always been the basis of making good medical decisions in the best interests of patients. The difference now is that it is the patient's assessment of this balance that matters rather than that of the physician. The balance depends on the magnitude and probability of the various benefits and burdens – when there is a high probability of great benefit it may be justified to accept considerable risk of harm. However, the reverse is also true, as was found when over 500 people were asked their treatment preferences if in coma with a small chance of complete recovery (see Table 6.2). Between 55% and 60% did not want life-prolonging treatment, presumably because they were unwilling to risk the possibility of surviving with severe brain damage. Similarly, most of a group of neurosurgeons wanted more than 90% probability of death or severe disability before they would withhold ventilation or surgery from a patient soon after severe head injury. Yet if they themselves were injured, three times as many surgeons would want treatment withheld at a much lower probability of a poor outcome (13). It seemed that they were not prepared to accept for themselves the level of risk of survival with severe brain damage that they would impose on their patients. Many commentators have stated that the only benefit that a permanently vegetative patient might gain from being kept alive is the very remote chance of limited late recovery, an outcome that is always associated with continuing very severe disability. Some opponents of withholding life-sustaining treatment quote this slight uncertainty to support their case. However, it seems clear that most patients and professionals do not look for an unrealistic degree of certainty before judging that the balance of benefits and burdens favours treatment withdrawal once a vegetative state has been declared permanent by the best criteria available.

Justice is perhaps the most difficult of the principles to apply in practice, but it is a useful reminder that it is both important and ethically acceptable to consider the wider repercussions for society of decisions made about individual patients. Gillon has suggested that three types of justice be recognized (7). There is the fair distribution of scarce resources (distributive justice), respect for peoples' rights (rights-based justice) and respect for morally acceptable laws (legal justice). Certainly permanently vegetative patients, who require 24 hours skilled nursing care, consume considerable resources. The Task Force estimated in 1994 that the total care costs for PVS patients in the US were in the range of $1–7 billion per year (14). Such expenditure without commensurate patient benefit could be regarded as a waste of resources on utilitarian principles, and indeed it has been suggested that a prudent allocator of health-care resources would give low priority to the care of these patients (15). In a survey of the attitudes of over 300 American physicians, 93% considered it ethical to discontinue payments for CPR, dialysis or transfusions for adults in a permanent vegetative state (16). Only 83% would stop payments for antibiotics and 76% for ANH. These same authors later suggested that PVS provided a paradigm for the rationing of health-care resources that should be acceptable to most physicians and citizens (17). An earlier proposal by Winslade (18) was that if termination of life-sustaining treatment for patients in PVS were to become the norm then the values of vitalists should be tolerated by encouraging them to seek continued care at their own expense. In the US scene, he suggested that this might be through paying supplemental premiums to private insurance companies to cover this particular eventuality. For the UK, Gillon (19) has suggested that treatment to prolong the lives of permanently vegetative patients should not be funded by the state.

Having described these four principles with some reference to their application to the management of permanently vegetative patients, it remains to deal with a number of controversies that persist in this difficult area of medical decision making. To some extent these have arisen because the development of decisions to limit some treatments for hopelessly ill patients initially applied to quite different types of situation. Acutely ill patients in intensive care were the first to give physicians cause to pause in their efforts to prolong the lives of the hopelessly ill. Such patients were without doubt terminally ill, had usually been treated only briefly in a fruitless attempt to save their lives, and it was not difficult to argue that to persist was futile and could deprive them of death with dignity. By 1990 it was found that almost half of all deaths in intensive care had followed a decision to withhold or withdraw treatment (20). Another group of patients eligible for limited treatment were seriously malformed infants and 2 years before *Quinlan* a medical journal had an article by a Jesuit on this topic under the title 'To save or let die: the dilemma of modern medicine' (21). More recently, concern has focused on the treatment of the demented elderly, another distinctly different group of patients. Meanwhile, the debate about euthanasia has sometimes obtruded on the issue of how to treat patients in PVS, with the concern that agreeing to let these patients die might result in a slippery slope to making euthanasia seem acceptable for other types of patient. In highlighting certain controversies, the considerable overlap and interaction between them will become obvious, and some arguments will begin to appear to be circular.

Sanctity versus quality of life

That biological life alone is not an unqualified good is widely accepted by many theologians, as already noted in Chapter 6. A Jesuit commentator has described the Judeo–Christian attitude thus: 'Life is indeed a basic and precious good, but a good to be preserved precisely as the condition of other values. These other values found the duty to preserve physical life and also dictate the limits of this duty' (21). These values are variously described as the ability to form relationships with other people, to decide and to act as a moral agent, and to gain some satisfaction from being alive. Because these values are not available to the vegetative patient some philosophers have argued that such a patient is no longer a person, and that because of this society does not owe that patient the same moral obligations as it does to conscious, cognitive human beings (p. 81). However, there are those who reject any attempt to judge the quality of life of others, while some assert that we fail in our duty of care if we do not make an attempt to do so for those unable to express their own views about themselves. Fortunately, there is an abundance of evidence as to how most people regard the quality of life in a permanent vegetative state (see Chapter 6), and the physician is not therefore relying on his own value judgement or that of the profession corporate when applying this consensus to an individual patient. There is of course a minority of vitalists who value life at any level, a view that denies both autonomy and the value of balancing benefits and burdens when deciding on what medical treatment for vegetative patients is appropriate or proportionate. The vitalist arguments were rejected unanimously by the Appleton conference (12).

Ordinary versus extraordinary treatments

Since the Pope's 1957 declaration that physicians are normally obliged to use only ordinary means to preserve life, there have been debates about how to distinguish these from extraordinary treatments. Initially ordinary was taken to mean generally available and widely used, whilst extraordinary would include advanced technological methods that were scarce and expensive. However, there has been a shift to including a reasonable likelihood of achieving a favourable outcome as part of the definition of ordinary treatment, and also to considering that unusual burdens incurred by a treatment, whether to the patient, his family or his carers, may justify calling a treatment extraordinary. In effect, this amounts to accepting the balance of benefits and burdens as a measure of what treatment is appropriate, and this is reflected in abandoning the ordinary/extraordinary dualism in favour of proportionate versus disproportionate treatment. This makes it more possible to concede that artificial nutrition and hydration may sometimes be disproportionate treatment, while many have found it difficult to regard it as extraordinary by the original definition. In the light of recent wide-ranging discussions about limiting treatment much less is now heard of ordinary vs. extraordinary treatments, which is regarded as more likely to confuse than to clarify matters.

Futility

Casual references to continued treatment of PVS patients as being futile were made in some of the early court cases. However, formal analysis of the concept of futility began with reactions to a proposal that CPR should be withheld from chronically demented patients without consulting relatives if the physician declared it to be a futile treatment (22). Schneiderman et al. (23) developed the notion that futility was the product of probability and utility, giving it a quantitative and qualitative component. They suggested that if a desired utility was not achieved in the last 100 cases it should be deemed quantitatively futile. In fact, this gives only 95% confidence that no more than three successes would occur in each subsequent 100 cases, which some consider makes this definition of futility too pessimistic. Utility can apply to a physiological effect, such as restarting the heart by CPR, or to overall patient benefit, such as duration and quality of life gained. Lack of utility (no physiological effect or a qualitatively poor result such as surviving in a vegetative state) would justify declaring life-prolonging treatment to be futile; and according to these authors such treatment need neither be offered nor even discussed with the patient or family members.

In a later paper, these authors acknowledged that this approach threatened to erode the gains in autonomy over paternalism that had occurred in recent years (24). This was because physicians were liable to use futility, as defined by them, as a trump card to ignore or overrule demands for certain treatments by patients or families. They maintained that physicians needed to adjust their values to reflect more closely those of society, while trying in discussions with families to reduce unrealistic expectations by providing reliable information about the likely outcomes associated with various treatment options. In this way, a family could form a view about what treatments they would regard as futile. While it has been stated that physicians have no duty to provide futile treatment, it has to be accepted that some families will challenge a medical view of futility. They will prefer to hold out hopes for a miracle, or will profess religious beliefs that prolonging life of any kind is an acceptable end in itself. Families of a permanently vegetative patient may even demand CPR (25). Providing treatment under these conditions may be against the ethic both of the individual physician and of the wider medical profession, who may argue that families should be able to choose only between effective treatments. Moreover, the physician's stewardship of society's resources should require wise choices in their use. However, this paper notes that, even in the absence of finding another physician willing to provide futile treatment, the tendency of courts in the US has been to respect the wishes of families (see the case of *Wanglie* p. 142).

Gillon (26) has suggested that futility is a term that should no longer be used because it is too ambiguous and pejorative, akin to the outmoded terms hysteric and hypochondriac. It is liable to produce hostility in discussions with families, because it implies that treating their relative is not judged worthwhile. It should be possible to discuss the realities of the situation sympathetically without using this word. The AMA has recently issued procedural guidelines for dealing with medical futility at the end of life (27). Although most previous discussions of futility have focused on whether or not to initiate CPR, this report puts continued treatment of permanently vegetative patients first in its list of futile treatments. It reiterates the need to avoid using futility as an excuse for not discussing management with the patient or family. Moreover, it cautions against the danger of using futility as a covert way to conserve resources. Indeed, studies have suggested that very modest savings would result from imposing earlier limits on treatment at the end of life, because for most conditions most medical costs have already been incurred by then. The AMA accepts that objectivity or consensus is difficult to attain when the issue is what constitutes 'worth-the-effort' quality of life. It suggests that institutions, such as hospitals, medical associations or religious bodies might develop standards to define proactively what interventions might be considered futile in defined circumstances. For example, an editorialist in the *New England Journal of Medicine* (28) suggested that it should be assumed that permanently vegetative patients would not want to be kept alive. This would shift the burden from those who now have to argue that further treatment is futile to those holding the idiosyncratic view that it is beneficial.

A philosopher has likewise argued that the default mode of modern medicine ought to be that, in the absence of any directives to the contrary, patients with specified neurological impairments would not receive life-sustaining treatment (29). If such a standard were accepted it would facilitate adoption of the AMA's suggestions for a fair process for negotiating about futility. Ideally this would begin with discussions with the patient or family before a crisis had occurred. Failing that, discussions would begin once a decision to limit treatment had become an option, with the offer of a second medical opinion if desired. If there was then a disagreement between the family and the physician, the help of the hospital ethics committee would be enlisted. Only if this did not resolve the issue, and attempts to transfer the patient to another physician or institution had been unsuccessful, would it be appropriate to consider going to court.

Withholding versus withdrawing

It is common clinical experience that physicians and nurses find it more difficult emotionally, if not rationally, to withdraw a treatment already started than to withhold it in the first place. When it comes to withdrawing, two-thirds of a group of American physicians with such a bias preferred withdrawing treatment that had been established for only a few days rather than for many months, although a third of this large sample had no preference (30). It is widely held, however, by philosophers and lawyers that there is no moral or legal distinction between withholding and withdrawing. In an investigation of nurses and doctors in the UK and the US, designed to see how closely these health professionals agreed with the views of ethicists, the greatest disagreement was on this question (31). Only 20% of UK and 34% of US health professionals agreed that withholding and withdrawing were equivalent. To suggest that the first is an omission and the second an action is also a false distinction based on the feeling that when death follows an action it may seem more culpable. What matters is the intention – in both cases it is to let nature takes its course. A philosophical case for regarding withdrawing as morally worse than withholding (32) has been refuted by Gillon (33).

In practice, treatment withdrawal is increasingly accepted as an aspect of compassionate clinical practice (34). In a report of deaths following limitation of treatment in two American intensive care units, withdrawals were four times more frequent than withholdings (20). This is not surprising because it is often only after a treatment has been tried and has proved unsuccessful that it can be declared futile. Withdrawing ANH from a vegetative patient can be regarded in this light, albeit the trial of treatment will have lasted for many months rather than the few hours or days of a trial of treatment in intensive care. Were withdrawal not regarded as an acceptable practice in medicine, there would be the risk that physicians might become reluctant in the acute stage to initiate some treatments that could be of benefit for fear that, if they proved ineffective, a prolonged period of futile treatment would be inevitable. In practical terms, it can be helpful when a specific treatment such as ANH is initiated to indicate to the treating team and the family that it would be for a trial period, after which the case for continuing it would be reviewed. This would also make it clear that consent to start treatment would not be taken to imply consent to continue it indefinitely after it had proved to have been ineffective.

The special problem of ANH

There have been numerous declarations that ANH should be regarded as medical treatment that can be discontinued when it is judged to be no longer of benefit to the patient. The President's Commission declared that, once the vegetative state was declared permanent, all life-sustaining therapies (including ANH) could be withdrawn (11). That same year (1983) saw the *Barber* court in California declare that ANH was medical treatment that could be withdrawn from a severely brain damaged patient (p. 000). This was reiterated by the *Conroy* court in New Jersey in 1985 (p. 000). Neither of these patients was vegetative and each of them died before the legal judgement was given so that the *Brophy* court in Massachusetts in 1986 was the first to authorize removal of ANH from a living patient who was permanently vegetative (p. 194). Many subsequent court decisions and a series of supporting statements from professional medical authorities on both sides of the Atlantic, have all maintained that ANH is similar to other treatments, such as a ventilator or dialysis, each of which replaces a lost physiological function, in this case swallowing.

In the survey of 500 people in Boston who were asked to imagine various future scenarios, as many said they would refuse ANH (80%) as would refuse CPR, major surgery, ventilation or dialysis (see Table 6.2). Yet in the European study of over 2000 physicians (35) fewer would ever consider withdrawing ANH from a patient in PVS (57%) than would withhold interventions for new complications (79%). When 450 American physicians were asked to list treatments in order of their willingness to withdraw them, their response was blood products, dialysis, vasopressors, parenteral nutrition, antibiotics, tube feeding and intravenous fluids (30). In both these examples of reluctance to withdraw ANH, most of the treatments that were more willingly foregone were in fact new interventions, and this may therefore reflect a greater willingness of physicians to withhold than to withdraw rather than to perceived differences between the various treatment modalities. A study in the Netherlands of over 5000 nonsudden deaths in hospitals, nursing homes and at home found that 30% followed a nontreatment decision (36). Withdrawals were as frequent as withholdings, and ANH was the treatment most commonly foregone, often for elderly demented patients.

Objectors to the withdrawal of ANH usually challenge the assertion that it is a form of medical treatment, regarding this declaration to be a device to allow it to be withdrawn by physicians when they consider it no longer of benefit. These critics prefer to regard ANH as an aspect of basic care that should be provided regardless of medical benefit. Some argue that ANH is not treatment because it does nothing to restore function or to heal diseased organs. However, that is true also of ventilation or dialysis which, like ANH, may be used temporarily until a critical failure of organ function recovers either spontaneously or in response to other medical interventions. If no such recovery occurs and the patient is either terminally ill or permanently unconscious these treatments, among others, are commonly withdrawn. Some patients who remain in permanent need of some of these types of technical support of lost function can live fulfilled lives, as can patients requiring drugs that replace deficient function such as diabetics taking insulin. No one would claim that this is not medical treatment because it replaces rather than restores a natural function.

Some argue that ANH differs from other treatments in that its denial always leads to death, whilst other modalities such as antibiotics and surgery may prove not to be as essential for prolongation of life as doctors withholding them believe them to be. However, that argument breaks down when applied to withdrawal of ventilation and dialysis from patients with apnoea or renal failure. A variant of this objection is to note the universality of the consequence of denying food and fluid, because it leads to death in healthy people as well as in patients with pathological conditions, an objection sometimes linked to references to planned deaths under oppressive political regimes (37). Another definition of medical treatment is that it requires medical skills for it to be delivered. Whilst critics concede that such skills are needed for placing or replacing gastric tubes they point out that the delivery of food and fluid is often done by families caring for vegetative patients at home. Others point out that some PVS patients can swallow small amounts slowly and that given enough time and effort their nutrition might be maintained without artificial or medical means. They regard ANH as a convenience rather than a necessity for such patients.

Those who maintain that ANH is part of basic care point to the symbolic significance of feeding the weak and vulnerable – infants, the acutely ill, the feeble elderly and the dying. This both shows compassion to them and expresses solidarity among human kind. Even for the dying patient, where many agree that feeding may not even contribute to comfort, families may insist that feeding should continue, and the patient's interests may then be sacrificed for the benefit of the family at the bedside. Stopping feeding may be seen as abandonment, but all withdrawal protocols emphasize the need to provide continuing comfort care and attention by nurses (38,39). There is also the emotive phrase 'starving to death' with the implication that denying ANH will lead to unpleasant symptoms and signs. That this sloganism of starvation is misleading has already been explained (p. 93), where the evidence for a peaceful and comfortable death even in those with some remaining consciousness is reviewed. The realities of tube feeding are far from the nurturing associated with assisting with natural feeding, and to persist with unwanted treatment that is without ultimate benefit to the patient can be seen as a poor way to show compassion. This point was emphasized by Gillick (40) when asserting that withholding ANH from patients with dementia was compatible with traditional Judaism. Indeed ANH might more truthfully be described as forced feeding, which sounds much less kind and compassionate.

It is important to recognize that permanently vegetative patients make up only a small minority of the patients for whom ANH is an option. Conscious, competent patients with advanced states of permanent paralysis may choose to forgo ANH (41,42). However, most of the estimated 250 000 on long-term ANH in the US are demented elderly patients. There is much discussion about the wisdom of withholding ANH from them when they get to the stage of refusing food, and also from elderly patients who have suffered a severe stroke as well as from other patients who are dying (43–47). Of 116 cases seeking guidance about ANH from the American Society for the Right to Die during 1985–90, only 15% were in a vegetative state compared with 70% of the 20 ANH cases coming to the courts in the same period (48). Only 35% of the vegetative cases were more than 70 years, compared with 79% of the other cases. Indeed the American Geriatric Society submitted a brief as *amicus curiae* to the US Supreme Court in the case of *Nancy Cruzan* in support of withdrawing ANH (49). It feared that if a distinction was made between nutritional support and other medical treatments so that its withdrawal was not allowed, there would be a profound impact on the care of many patients, especially the elderly. It would then be impossible, it maintained, 'to sustain a patient-centered standard of medical decision-making and the maximisation of life extension would be required without regard to the suffering thereby imposed'. An opposing view was expressed in a brief to the same court from a number of associations representing people with disabilities, their families and the professionals who served them (50). Their fear was that if the court decided to allow withdrawal of ANH from *Nancy Cruzan* this would jeopardize the lives and well-being of many vulnerable people in the country. This claim for the danger of a slippery slope had been specifically rejected some years previously in a commentary on the *Brophy* case (51).

The reluctance on the part of some to accept that ANH can be withdrawn as readily as other life-prolonging treatments may derive in part from the fact that this withdrawal could apply to so many more patients than the limited number whose lives depend on high technology medical treatments. The possibility of abuse therefore seems greater, and some states in America that accepted treatment refusals from living wills or surrogates did not at first allow withdrawal of ANH. However, since the *Cruzan* case many of these statutes have been amended to allow withdrawal from permanently unconscious patients (which include those in PVS). In Britain, court approval is still required before withdrawing ANH from a patient in PVS. For patients who are not vegetative, the BMA has issued guidance suggesting additional procedural safeguards for decisions to withdraw ANH when death is not imminent and the patient's wishes are not known (52). These would require a second senior medical opinion to be obtained and recorded, and that medical notes be kept for subsequent review to confirm that the decision had been appropriate. More than one English judge has suggested the minor verbal adjustment of regarding ANH as part of medical **care**. This would still allow justification for its use to depend on the balance of benefits and burdens. Whilst ANH may impose actual experienced burdens on patients with residual consciousness, who may try to pull out nasogastric tubes, this does not apply to the vegetative patient. Nor can it be claimed that ANH itself is a significant financial burden. It is the continuing total care that is expensive, and it is the totality of continued vegetative existence that is, in the eyes of most people, the burden resulting from persisting with ANH. What should determine whether or not to continue treatment with ANH is therefore how those involved regard the prolongation of life in a permanent vegetative state. Lack of benefit will always be a stronger argument than the burden of continuing treatment.

The Catholic Church

Ambivalence is the feature of the reaction of this church to the problem of the permanently vegetative patient over the years. The local Catholic bishops supported the removal of the respirator in the *Quinlan* case, while the Vatican was later to harass the parents for their stance (pp. 98, 188). The petitioner for the removal of the respirator in the *Fox* case (53) was the religious superior of the vegetative patient. In the case of *Conroy* (p. 192), who was demented but not in PVS, the bishops also supported the withdrawal of ANH. The following year in the case of *Brophy* (p. 194), who was also a practising Catholic, there was conflicting advice from the clergy. However, in a vegetative case the same year, the bishops declared that Catholic patients and their families and caregivers were obliged to accept, or to continue if once begun, artificial medical measures that provided nutrition and hydration. To anticipate any special pleading they stated that this would apply regardless of the medical condition, the stated wishes of the patient or family, or the suffering or other burdens resulting from continued life. This inconsistency of the bishops was explored in some detail in an article by two American Jesuits (54). They robustly challenged this most recent declaration, quoting other Catholic authorities. These included the statement of another Jesuit that no remedy is obligatory unless it offers a reasonable hope of checking or curing a disease, and that all artificial means of sustaining life are remedies for some diseased or defective condition. It seemed to them that it was fear of euthanasia that led the bishops to their uncompromising position. They concluded that 'to count mere vegetative existence as a benefit to patients was to let slip one's grasp on the heart of Catholic tradition in this matter'.

Since then there has been acceptance of the withdrawal of ANH by many individual Catholics, including priests, but others have put a contrary view. Some Catholic hospitals in the US have adopted a policy of not allowing the withdrawal of ANH even if legally sanctioned, making patient transfer necessary if the wishes of the family and the court are to be met. The issues behind these differing opinions are well set out in the statements of the Committee for Pro-life Activities of the National Conference of Catholic Bishops in the US. These lengthy pronouncements appeared in 1992 (55) and in 1999 (56). Each of them admitted that some Catholics strongly disagreed on how to apply agreed moral principles to patients, and that the church's teaching authority had failed to resolve these differences. It needs a keen eye to detect any substantial difference between these two declarations, each of which concluded with the same disclaimer – 'This document is our first word and not our last word on this subject'.

Killing or letting die

In this controversy it is particularly difficult to separate the ethical and legal approaches. The accepted practice of forgoing life-prolonging treatments emerged in the context of terminally ill patients, as already explained. Many such patients were in intensive care, expected to die within hours, days or weeks even with continuing treatment. However, 'terminal' came later to be variously defined as an expectation of life of several months up to a year, while some preferred a less restrictive definition such as irrecoverable or irreversible, regardless of duration of survival. None the less, a problem was perceived in applying a practice originally developed for those who were acutely and terminally ill to PVS patients, who had been ill for months or years and could live for several more years if life-sustaining treatment was maintained. Some American recommendations (and some courts) have specifically exempted PVS patients from the need to have a limited life expectation before withdrawing life-sustaining treatment, pointing to the paradox that the longer that nonbeneficial treatment is likely to continue, the greater the potential harm to the patient. This did not assuage some critics who insisted that the inevitable early death of a patient who could have lived for years meant that those who had stopped ANH had killed the patient. The counter argument was that patients in PVS were already in a dying process that had been temporarily halted by ANH, the withdrawal of which simply allowed this process to be resumed. This argument regarded ANH as a trial of treatment that had proved ineffective. Some might even claim that as brain death was regarded as an unnatural artifact made possible by the ventilator, so the vegetative state might be considered to be an artificial state produced by medical intervention. In both instances the cause of death when treatment was withdrawn was widely agreed in legal circles to have been the original brain damage, not suffocation or starvation. It would be patently absurd to regard every death following the withdrawal of ineffective treatment as the result of the doctor having killed the patient.

Utilitarians maintain that a strong moral prohibition against killing reduces harm, whilst such an objection to letting die would cause much more harm and bring much less benefit overall (57). Indeed, respect for autonomy implies that there are circumstances where it is not only permissible but required that the physician let the patient die, as when a patient has refused life-prolonging treatment. Some aspects of how to respect the autonomy of the incompetent patient have already been discussed (p. 101), and this problem has led to varying legal solutions in different countries (see Chapters 9, 10, 11).

Another argument depends on the perceived difference between acts and omissions although in most situations these are seen as morally equivalent, other things being equal (57,58). Indeed, the physician who decides to omit treatment is still acting as a moral agent. However, if the physician were to give a PVS patient a lethal injection the death could no longer be regarded as natural, but the result of active intervention. Yet the legal and moral differences between these acts and omissions are open to argument (59,60).

The law makes much of intention, as do Catholic theologians (56,57). Defenders of treatment withdrawal maintain that death is a foreseen but not intended consequence of a decision to withdraw nonbeneficial or unwanted treatment. It might even be argued as an example of the doctrine of double effect, more often applied to drugs given to relieve symptoms but which may hasten death. Others maintain that as the rationale for stopping ANH is that life in PVS is not a benefit, and that as death is such an inevitable consequence, it is naive to pretend that the patient's death was not intended. Indeed the phrase to 'let die' leaves no doubt about the intention. Motive is not the same as intention – the good motives of those accused of active 'mercy' killings do not prevent them facing criminal charges and being convicted, although their motives often result in mitigating the sentence passed.

Some international variations

Britain

Doctors in Britain have been more reluctant than those in America to accept a formal approach to treatment-limiting decisions. It has already been noted that in 1970 the *Lancet* did not respond sympathetically to pleas for doctors to recognize when patients should be let die (p. 73). Yet by that time the first hospice had already been opened in London, pioneering an approach to the care of terminally ill cancer patients that was based on accepting that the time for active curative or even palliative treatment of the cancer had passed. Continuing care would thenceforth be confined to relieving symptoms and attending to the dying patient's immediate needs, both physical and spiritual. In 1982, an editorial by a prominent London physician deplored the American approach of formal protocols for limiting treatment (61). Interestingly, his title 'Thou shalt not strive officiously' was a misquotation of an early Victorian poet's couplet 'Thou shalt not kill; but need'st not strive/ Officiously to keep alive'. He implied that the need for rules to deal with the problem of doctors persisting with inappropriate, aggressive treatment of terminally ill patients was largely an American one. He maintained that the extent of medical litigation in America had led to an atmosphere of hostility towards, and even mistrust of, physicians. He concluded 'There seems no call for such measures in Britain where the medical team is under few constraints – familial, ethical, and, least of all, legal – to act as it sees fit in the best interests of the patient'. It was not until 1989 that another commentator, referring to US government-sponsored protocols for decisions about life-sustaining treatments, suggested that 'learning from America' might be wise (62), and it was another 10 years before the BMA published its guidelines on withholding and withdrawing treatment (52).

Discussion in Britain about limiting life-prolonging treatment of patients in the vegetative state has been considerably influenced by the apparent association of this with euthanasia. The question of legalizing euthanasia has been on the medico-political agenda in Britain since 1935, when a number of eminent physicians formed the Voluntary Euthanasia Society, since when the matter has been debated in Parliament on at least five occasions. Yet it was in the BMA report on Euthanasia in 1988, which was categorically against any change in the law that forbids euthanasia, that the first formal statement about the appropriateness of withdrawing treatment (including ANH) from vegetative patients appeared (63). It was, however, only the condemnation of euthanasia that attracted attention in the public and medical press and the aside about vegetative patients passed unnoticed. However, the BMA consultation paper on the treatment of vegetative patients in September 1992, shortly before the *Bland* case came to court, referred repeatedly to the previous Euthanasia Report in support of its conclusion that withdrawal of ANH was appropriate (64).

In 1991, the majority of a working party of the Institute of Medical Ethics concluded that withdrawal of ANH was morally justified, and urged more professional bodies to recognize this publicly (65). The remit of this working party was 'The ethics of prolonging life and assisting death', and in a report the previous year it had argued that it was sometimes ethically justified to assist the death of a patient (66). Again, therefore, treatment withdrawal from vegetative patients might appear to be linked to euthanasia. This association was reinforced by the chance that only 8 weeks before the *Bland* case came to court in London in November 1992 the High Court there had convicted *Dr Cox*, a hospital consultant, of attempted murder for giving a fatal injection to a terminally ill patient in great pain.

One consequence of these two trials was that the House of Lords was required to set up a select committee on medical ethics which was charged with reviewing the public policy issues associated with both euthanasia and the withdrawal of treatment from vegetative patients. Its report (67) gained most attention for its rejection of any relaxation of the law against euthanasia. As for the vegetative state, its conclusions were singularly unhelpful but fortunately they appear to have had no effect on medical or legal practice (p. 153).

Judges, other legal commentators and moralists have echoed American opinion by repeatedly stating that withdrawal of nonbeneficial treatment that leads to death cannot be equated with euthanasia. Following extensive debate in the print and broadcast media there is general acceptance by the public of the principle of treatment withdrawal. However, some who are particularly fearful of any development in medical practice that might seem to begin a slippery slope towards acceptance of euthanasia have objected to withdrawal of ANH from PVS patients. Indeed, when the BMA in 1999 published its guidance on limiting life-prolonging treatment (including ANH) from both vegetative and other patients (p. 112), this attempt to reassure the public by formalizing what was already accepted practice led to some adverse comment. Some regarded it as a move towards involuntary euthanasia, and one MP introduced into Parliament a Medical Treatment (prevention of euthanasia) Bill to outlaw withdrawing ANH even from vegetative patients. After some debate in early 2000, however, this bill was dropped before getting as far as a vote. Another attempt to challenge the practice of treatment withdrawal from vegetative patients was mounted later that year by the antieuthanasia pressure group ALERT (Against Legalized Euthanasia – Research and Testing). Its attempt to put the case in a court deciding about two vegetative patients that withdrawal of ANH was against the Human Rights Act was disallowed by the judge. She later ruled that this Act did not affect the status quo in regard to giving legal approval of withdrawal of ANH from patients in a permanent vegetative state (p. 162). Reluctance to confront the euthanasia issue is claimed to have led to unhelpful legal approaches to the problem of PVS in Britain (pp. 166, 167).

As in the US, Catholic opinion in the UK has been divided. Two separate comments in a leading Catholic journal (*The Tablet*) soon after the *Bland* case accepted that withdrawal of ANH from vegetative patients was compatible with Catholic tradition (68,69). Yet the decision was condemned as euthanasia in a statement from the bishops of England and Wales (70). Later comment from a Catholic academic lawyer was very critical of the *Bland* decision (71) and another consistent critic has been the director of the Catholic Linacre Centre (72). In the book *Euthanasia Examined*, edited by another Catholic academic lawyer, both the above authors had chapters (73), and indeed the *Bland* case was referred to in all but five of the 18 chapters, and one of those five referred to *Cruzan*. The theme was that the *Bland* decision appeared to authorize euthanasia and/or physician-assisted suicide – both of which are anathema to the Catholic Church.

However, in the Republic of Ireland, where 91% of the population are Catholic, the High Court in 1995 heard conflicting views from different church authorities but decided to allow ANH to be withdrawn from a 45-year-old woman who had been vegetative for 23 years (p. 214).

Scandinavia

An international meeting in Italy in 1994 recorded that treatment withdrawal without reference to the courts had become accepted practice in Norway, Sweden and Denmark (74). This appeared to have developed in the light of general statements about discontinuing nonbeneficial treatments at the end of life, which did not include specific reference to the vegetative state.

Belgium

In 1992 the Bioethics Committee of the Catholic University of Leuven published a statement recommending treatment withdrawal (including ANH) from patients in a permanent vegetative state, without reference to the courts (75). This appears to have become accepted practice in Belgium, although in the European study only 56% of Belgian doctors would consider withdrawing ANH (35).

Netherlands

The Netherlands Health Council produced a long document on the management of vegetative patients in 1994 (76). It accepted that tube feeding was medical treatment and recommended its withdrawal 6 months after anoxic damage and 12 months after head injury, without involvement of the courts. Vegetative patients were not eligible for euthanasia as they could not fulfil the requirement that patients themselves must request this. The frequency of decisions to forgo treatment from patients in general in the Netherlands, and that withdrawing ANH is common practice, has already been noted (p. 34). In the European study, 70% of doctors in the Netherlands would consider withdrawing ANH, the next highest after the 73% in the UK (35).

Germany

By reason of memories of the Nazi era, there is great reluctance to take decisions to allow the early death of patients whose quality of life is deemed 'not worthwhile'. This was the phrase used to justify euthanasia for mentally disabled and other groups in the 1930s, well before the development of death camps. There is a well-organized lobby in Germany protecting the rights of vegetative patients to continued treatment, and the survey of doctors' views about treatment (35) found many fewer (16%) willing to consider withdrawing ANH than in most other European countries (average 57%). However, the courts have approved such withdrawal when it could be shown to reflect the presumed will of the patient (p. 179).

France

In a long discussion of the ethical treatment of vegetative patients, Lamau et al. (77) pointed out that, although most such patients in France were in one of a small number of specialist units, their long-term care did pose ethical and economic problems. They emphasized that there was not the same regard for patient autonomy as in Anglo-American societies. Although French doctors were now more likely than formerly to listen to the patient's point of view they retained the right to make decisions for their patients – described as moderate paternalism. Although the law recognized the right of the patient to refuse treatment the doctor was more likely to respond that his duty of care to a fellow human being was more important, and this was usually taken to involve the continuation of nursing care, including ANH. Although there was brief mention of the possibility of withdrawing ANH to let the patient die, the implication was that this would hardly ever be contemplated, for fear that it be labelled passive euthanasia. However, a large group of French hospital doctors has recently declared their support for withholding and withdrawing treatment in intensive care, and their report indicated that they practiced what they preached (p. 181). There was reluctance on the part of the French doctors to participate in the European survey (35) and of the small number who did respond only 14% were willing ever to consider withdrawal of ANH. However, 78% would consider withholding interventions for new complications.

Italy

A somewhat similar attitude appears to apply in Italy (78). The concept of 'worse than death' is challenged, as is the futility of continuing with ANH and the wisdom of immediately acting on an advance directive that would result in letting the patient die. Whilst there will usually be a presumption to continue treatment, it is accepted as legitimate to have rules about when to let die, in order to avoid 'vitalist obstinacy'. It seems, however, to be implied that only when there was an advance directive would withdrawal of ANH be regarded as not morally objectionable.

Southern European countries

Two articles from Spain, one on advance directives (79) with only a passing mention of patients with irreversible unconsciousness, the other on bioethics in general (80), contrast the US with three European traditions – Anglo-Saxon, North European and Mediterranean. In the last of these, which is Catholic, there is less tendency for patients and their families to regard themselves as consumers, distrustful of doctors and keen on strict procedures. Nor is secular moralism, with its ideology of liberalism, privacy and autonomy, so dominant. Virtue is more highly prized than rights, justice than autonomy, stoicism than utilitarianism. Statutory law is the rule rather than the accumulated decisions about individuals that characterize common law jurisdictions. With less concern for individual choice there is more trust in family support and in the advice of doctors, and it is more likely that treatment will be demanded than its withdrawal discussed or requested. Greece was the only Mediterranean country included in the European survey (35) and only 23% of doctors there were willing to consider withdrawing ANH. What was surprising was that even fewer (21%) would consider withholding treatment for complications, far lower than the next lowest country, which was Germany, where 58% were willing to do this.

New Zealand

The Medical Council of New Zealand commissioned a report on the withdrawal of ANH from permanently vegetative patients from the Bioethics Research Centre at the University of Otago. The report came in

February 1993, before the *Bland* case was completed (81). Relying on this source the New Zealand Medical Association produced a policy document on the vegetative state in 1994 (82). This declared that it was appropriate to discontinue ANH once the treating doctor and one other doctor considered the vegetative state to be permanent, usually a period of several months. It stated that recourse to a court of law was undesirable unless there was a specific issue of dispute.

REFERENCES

1 Pius XII. Pope speaks on prolongation of life. *Osservatore Romano* 1957; 4: 393–8

2 Ad hoc committee of the Harvard Medical School. A definition of irreversible coma. *JAMA* 1968; 205: 85–8

3 Cassem NH. Confronting the decision to let death come. *Crit Care Med* 1974; 2: 113–17

4 *In re Quinlan.* 70.NJ 10 355 A2d 647 (1976)

5 American Medical Association. Standards for cardiopulmonary resuscitation (CPR) and emergency cardiac care (ECC) v medical considerations and recommendations. *JAMA* 1974; 227: Suppl 864–6

6 Beauchamp TL, Childress JF. *Principles of biomedical ethics.* Oxford University Press, New York, 1979

7 Gillon RA. The Four Principles revisited – a reappraisal. In *Principles of Health Care Ethics* (chapter 28). Chichester: John Wiley & Sons, 1994: 319–34

8 Beauchamp TL. The 'Four Principles' approach. In *Principles of Health Care Ethics* (chapter 1) Gillon RA (Ed). Chichester: John Wiley & Sons, 1994: 3–12

9 Mill JS. *On Liberty*, Warnock M (Ed). London: Collins Fontana Library, 1962

10 Justice Cardozo. In *Schloendorff* v *Society of New York Hospitals.*(1914) 211 NY 125.105 NE 92–3

11 President's Commission for the Study of Ethical Problems in Medicine. *Deciding to forego life-sustaining treatment.* Washington DC, US Government Printing Office, 1983

12 Stanley JM. The Appleton International Conference. Developing guidelines for decisions to forgo life-prolonging medical treatment. *J Med Ethics* 1992; 18: Suppl 1–23

13 Barlow P, Teasdale G. Prediction of outcome and the management of severe head injuries: the attitudes of neurosurgeons. *Neurosurgery* 1986; 19: 989–91

14 The Multi-Society Task Force on the persistent vegetative state. Statement on medical aspects of the persistent vegetative state. *N Engl J Med* 1994; 330: 1572–9

15 Brock DW. Justice and the severely demented elderly. *J Med Philos* 1988; 13: 73–99

16 Payne K, Taylor RM, Stocking C et al. Physicians' attitudes about the care of patients in the persistent vegetative state: a national survey. *Ann Intern Med* 1996; 125: 104–10

17 Payne SK, Taylor RM. The persistent vegetative state and anencephaly: problematic paradigms for discussing futility and rationing. *Sem Neurology* 1997; 17: 257–63

18 Winslade WJ. Permanently unconscious patients: a radical proposal. *Tex Med* 1993; 89: 16

19 Gillon R. Persistent vegetative state and withdrawal of nutrition and hydration. *J Med Ethics* 1993; 19: 67–8

20 Smedira NG, Evans BH, Grais US et al. Withholding and withdrawing of life support from the critically ill. *N Engl J Med* 1990; 322: 309–15

21 McCormick RA. To save or let die: the dilemma of modern medicine. *JAMA* 1974; 229: 172–6

22 Youngner SA. Who defines futility? *JAMA* 1988; 260: 2094–5

23 Schneiderman LJ, Jecker NS, Jonsen AR. Medical futility: its meaning and ethical implications. *Ann Intern Med* 1990; 112: 949–54

24 Schneiderman LJ, Faber-Langendoen K, Jecker NS. Beyond futility to an ethic of care. *Am J Med* 1994; 96: 110–4

25 Weijer C. Cardiopulmonary resuscitation for patients in a persistent vegetative state: futile or acceptable? *CAMJ* 1998; 158: 491–3

26 Gillon R. 'Futility' – too ambiguous and pejorative a term. *J Med Ethics* 1997; 23: 339–40

27 Council on Ethical and Judicial Affairs, American Medical Association. Medical futility in end-of-life care. *JAMA* 1999; 281: 937–41

28 Angell M. After Quinlan: the dilemma of the persistent vegetative state. *N Engl J Med* 1994; 330: 1524–5

29 Thomasma DC. Surrogate decisions at risk. *J Am Geriatr Soc* 1990; 38: 603–4

30 Christakis NA, Asch DA. Biases in how physicians choose to withdraw life-support. *Lancet* 1993; 342: 642–6

31 Dickenson DL. Are medical ethicists out of touch? Pracitioner attitudes in the US and the UK towards decisions at the end of life. *J Med Ethics* 2000; 26: 254–60

32 Sulmasy D, Sugarman J. Are withdrawing and withholding therapy always morally equivalent? *J Med Ethics* 1994; 20: 218–22

33 Gillon R. Withholding and withdrawing life-prolonging treatment – moral implications of a thought experiment. *J Med Ethics* 1994; 20: 203–4

34 Brody H, Campbell, ML Faber-Langendoen et al. Withdrawing intensive life-sustaining treatment – recommendations for compassionate clinical management. *N Engl J Med* 1997; 336: 652–7

35 Grubb A, Walsh P, Lambe N et al. *The moral and legal issues surrounding the treatment and care of patients in persistent vegetative state.* Report to European

Biomedical and Health Research Programme, 1997 [on file in the Library of the Centre of Medical Ethics, King's College, London]

36 Groenwoud JH, van der Heide A, Kester JGC et al. A nationwide study of decisions to forego life-prolonging treatment in Dutch medical practice. *Arch Intern Med.* 2000; 160: 357–63

37 Derr PG. Why food and fluids can never be denied. *Hastings Cent Report* 1986; Feb: 28–30

38 American Nursing Association. *Position statement: foregoing nutrition and hydration.* 1992; April

39 Ohlenberg E. We withdraw nutrition – not care. *RN* 1996; May: 36–40

40 Gillick MR. Artificial nutrition and hydration in the patient with advanced dementia: is withholding treatment compatible with traditional Judaism? *J Med Ethics* 2001; 27: 12–15

41 American Academy of Neurology. Position statement: certain aspects of the care and management of profoundly and irreversibly paralysed patients with retained consciousness and cognition. *Neurology* 1993; 43: 222–3

42 Bernat JL, Cranford RE, Kittredge FI et al. Competent patients with advanced states of permanent paralysis have the right to forgo life-sustaining therapy. *Neurology* 1993; 43: 224–5

43 Campbell-Taylor I, Fisher RH. The clinical case against tube feeding in palliative care of the elderly. *J Am Geriatr Soc* 1987; 35: 1100–104

44 Printz LA. Terminal dehydration: a compassionate treatment. *Arch Intern Med* 1992; 125: 104–10

45 Sullivan RJ. Accepting death without artificial nutrition or hydration. *J Gen Intern Med* 1993; 8: 220–24

46 Lennard-Jones JE. Giving or witholding fluid and nutrients: ethical and legal aspects. *J R Coll Physicians Lond* 1999; 33: 39–45

47 Gillick MR. Rethinking the role of tube feeding in patients with advanced dementia. *N Engl J Med* 2000; 342: 206–10

48 Ahronheim JC, Mulvihill M. Refusal of tube feeding as seen from a patient advocacy organisation: a comparison with landmark court cases. *J Am Geriatr Soc* 1991; 39: 1124–7

49 Glover JJ. The case of Ms Cruzan and the care of the elderly. *J Am Geriatr Soc* 1990; 38: 588–93

50 Bopp J, Marzen TJ, Nimz MM et al. Abridged brief as *Amici Curiae* of the Association for Retarded Citizens of the United States et al. (in case of *Cruzan*). *J Am Geriatr Soc* 1990; 38: 580–87

51 Steinbrook R, Lo B. Artificial feeding – solid ground, not slippery slope. *N Engl J Med* 1988; 318: 286–90

52 British Medical Association. *Withholding or withdrawing life-prolonging medical treatment: guidance for decision-making.* London: BMJ Books. 1999

53 McCormick RJ. The Fox case. *JAMA* 1980; 244: 2165–6

54 Paris JJ, McCormick RA. The Catholic tradition on the use of nutrition and fluids. *America* 1987; 2 May: 356–61

55 Committee for Pro-life Activities of the National Conference of Catholic Bishops in the US Nutrition and hydration: moral and pastoral reflections. *Issues Law Med* 1992; 6: 359–62

56 Committee for Pro-life Activities of the National Conference of Catholic Bishops in the US. Nutrition and hydration: moral and pastoral reflections. *J Contemp Health Law Policy* 1999; 15: 455–77

57 Gillon R. Acts and omissions: killing and letting die. *J Med Ethics* 1984; 2: 59–60, 72

58 Gillon R. Euthanasia, withholding life-prolonging treatment, and moral differences between killing and letting die. *J Med Ethics* 1988; 14: 115–17

59 Ferguson PR. Causing death or allowing to die; developments in the law. *J Med Ethics* 1997; 23: 368–72

60 Randall F. Why causing death is not necessarily morally equivalent to allowing to die – a response to Ferguson. *J Med Ethics* 1997; 23: 373–6

61 Bayliss RIS. Thou shalt not strive officiously. *BMJ* 1982; 285: 1373–5

62 Williams BT. Life-sustaining technology: making the decisions. *BMJ* 1989; 98: 978

63 Working Party of the British Medical Association. *The euthanasia report.* London: BMA, 1988

64 Medical Ethics Committee of the British Medical Association. *Discussion paper on treatment of patients in the persistent vegetative state.* London: BMA, 1992

65 Institute of Medical Ethics Working Party. Withdrawal of life-support from patients in a persistent vegetative state. *Lancet* 1991; 337; 96–8

66 Institute of Medical Ethics Working Party. Assisted death. *Lancet* 1990; 336: 610–13

67 House of Lords. *Report of select committee on medical ethics.* HL 21–1. London: HMSO, 1994

68 McQueen M, Walsh JL. Comment on the *Bland* case. *The Tablet* 1992; 19/26 December

69 Kelly K. Comment on the *Bland* case. *The Tablet* 1993; 13 March

70 Budd C. *Euthanasia and hard cases.* London: Catholic Media Office, 1992

71 Finnis JM. *Bland*: crossing the Rubicon? *Law Q Rev* 1993; 109; 329–37

72 Gormally L. Definitions of personhood: implications for the care of PVS patients. *Ethics Med* 1993; 9: 44–8

73 Keown J (Ed). *Euthanasia examined: ethical, clinical and legal perspectives.* Cambridge: Cambridge University Press, 1995

74 Winslade WJ. Permanently unconscious patients: the need for responsible medical, legal, and public policies. Unpublished report of international conference in Bellagio, Italy. 1994

75 Katholicke Universiteit Leuven Research Committee on Medical Ethics. Ethical considerations on the persistent vegetative state. *Ethischee Perspect* 1992; 2: 14–16

76 Health Council of the Netherlands Committee on Vegetative State. *Patients in a Vegetative State*. The Hague: Health Council of the Netherlands, 1994

77 Lamau M-L, Cadore B, Boitte P. From the ethical treatment of patients in a persistent vegetative state to a philosophical reflection on contemporary medicine. *Theor Med* 1997; 18: 237–62

78 Cattorini, P Reichlin M. Persistent vegetative state: a presumption to treat. *Theor Med* 1997; 18: 263–81

79 Sanchez-Gonzalez MA. Advance directives outside the USA: are they the best solution everywhere? *Theor Med* 1997; 18: 282–301

80 Gracia D. The intellectual basis of bioethics in Southern European countries. *Bioethics* 1993; 7: 97–107

81 Bioethics Research Centre, University of Otago. *Persistent vegetative state and the withdrawal of food and fluids*. Report for the Medical Council of New Zealand, February 1993

82 New Zealand Medical Association Public Issues Advisory Committee. *Policy Paper: Persistent Vegetative State*. Wellington: New Zealand Medical Association, 1994

9

Legal issues in the United States

The law came late on the scene of medical decision making about patients who were considered to be hopelessly ill and unable to benefit from further medical intervention. However, with the *Quinlan* case in 1976 it came much sooner in the US than in England, where the first vegetative case (*Bland*) did not come until 16 years later. The legal arguments raised by withdrawing treatment from vegetative patients had therefore been exhaustively rehearsed in courts and commentaries in the US before other jurisdictions faced this problem. Inevitably, therefore, the American experience influenced how others later approached this issue.

The New Jersey court broke new legal ground in 1976 when it ruled that withdrawing life-sustaining treatment from *Karen Quinlan*, who was vegetative, was a matter to be decided by her family in consultation with her physicians (1). The court acknowledged that it had already become accepted good medical practice to limit life-prolonging treatment in terminal cases when there seemed to be a conflict between two duties of a physician – to prolong life and to prevent suffering (p. 187). However, the court pointed out that, so far, this had been happening without the sanction of civil law. The importance of involving the law was to give the approval of society to this medical practice and to suggest due process for physicians and families in these sensitive situations. Giving formal legitimacy to such practice should have reassured physicians, who had hitherto been overly cautious about discontinuing nonbeneficial treatment, that they had the protection of the law. In turn, that should have given more patients protection from unwanted treatment when fear of litigation was the real reason for continued treatment, rather than a convenient excuse for the physician's reluctance to accept that his interventions were no longer benefiting the patient.

The *Quinlan* case prompted three papers in the New England Journal of Medicine later that same year. The first, on optimum care for hopelessly ill patients, was from the Clinical Care Committee of the Massachusetts General Hospital (2). The second was on orders not to resuscitate (3), expanding on an earlier statement from the AMA. The third was on living wills (4), proposals for which had first been published in 1969. An editorial comment by a lawyer applauded hospitals for 'coming out of the closet' about terminating life support, which had already become common practice (5), but this commentator wished that there had been more clarity in these three papers about who was supposed to benefit from these statements. Was it patients anxious to be free from the tyranny of a technologic imperative, or was it society concerned to avoid the burden and expense of caring for a growing multitude of extravagantly demanding moribund persons?

Noting that lawyers had contributed to all three papers, he predicted that it was likely that more cases would soon be taken to court, even though the final *Quinlan* judgement had recommended that such decisions should be the business only of physicians and families. This prediction was fulfilled, for between 1977 and 1990 there were 49 cases in State courts and one in the US Supreme Court seeking permission to limit life-prolonging treatment, 27 of them for vegetative patients, ten for other incompetent patients and 13 for competent patients (6). The importance of decisions about these other types of patient was that the ethical and legal principles applied to them influenced the approach to vegetative patients. The next five cases through the courts were all acutely ill patients expected soon to die and the treatments dealt with were ventilators, DNR orders, dialysis or chemotherapy. Many of these terminally ill patients were conscious and suffering and competent to request that treatment be limited. The problem of applying this practice to vegetative patients was that their death was not imminent, that they were not suffering and that they could not participate in decision making. Indeed it was 10 years after *Quinlan* before the case of *Brophy* (p. 194), the first time an American court authorized withdrawing feeding from a living vegetative patient (7).

Reasons for allowing treatment withdrawal

These may be regarded as preserving a number of rights that a person can expect to have respected in a Western democracy.

Right to autonomy

Whilst this is considered the most important of the ethical principles underlying medical practice (p. 99) it is also well-established in law. In the New York Court of Appeals in 1914, Judge Cardozo declared 'Every human being of adult years and sound mind has a right to determine what should be done with his own body' (8). This is embodied in the legal principle of consent, which makes it a battery and a trespass for a doctor to do anything to a patient without his consent. In legal terms, this can be considered to be the common law right to self-determination.

The law is clear that a patient may not only withhold consent for a new intervention but may also withdraw consent for the continuation of treatment already started. Nor need any convincing reasons for refusal be given, and even a physician who considers the patient's decision unwise must comply with it, provided that the patient is considered to be competent and has been fully informed of the consequences of refusing treatment. The presumption is that the patient has weighed the balance between the expected, or at least perceived, benefits and burdens of the proposed treatment and has decided that it is not in his best interests to agree to its initiation or continuation. This has been the reason for several courts having agreed to requests from competent patients to abandon feeding or ventilator support, most of them having had severe progressive or permanent paralysis (e.g amyotrophic lateral sclerosis, locked-in syndrome or high spinal cord injury).

The right to refuse life-sustaining treatment is not absolute, however. Four possible countervailing interests of society are to preserve life, to prevent suicide, to safeguard the integrity of the medical profession and to protect innocent third parties (such as relatives whose inheritance might be at risk from a decision to allow earlier death). The court decisions that have allowed competent patients to have life-sustaining treatment stopped imply that the state does not claim an unqualified interest in the preservation of life, but that it allows that the quality of that life, particularly as judged by the patient, is a relevant factor. None the less, State Attorneys General have often opposed treatment withdrawal in these cases, arguing that the state does have an overriding interest in the preservation of life. Some have expressed concern that if it were agreed to allow a particular patient to die there would be a danger of eroding respect for life in other situations – the slippery slope argument.

As for suicide, it is argued that the intention of the patient refusing treatment is not to die but to be free of burdensome interventions, and numerous courts have asserted that refusal of treatment should not be construed as suicide. Indeed, the irrelevance of suicide is a central feature of the Natural Death Statutes enacted by many states, following California's example in 1976. It is, therefore, unwise to equate the right to refuse treatment with a right to die, a phrase often adopted by the media. Rather, it is an aspect of the right to choose how to live one's life.

As for the integrity of the medical profession, it is generally agreed that physicians have a duty to respect their patients' preferences, and that they do not have a duty to provide treatment that does not benefit a patient. Regarding the specific problem of vegetative patients there have been several position statements from professional medical organizations, such as the AMA and those representing intensivists and neurologists, stating that treatment withdrawal is part of good medical practice. Sometimes an individual physician or the institution in which he works objects to a court-approved decision to limit treatment, maintaining that their autonomy is infringed by requiring them to comply. Again, the courts have been clear in their response to such objections – the patient should be transferred to another physician or institution that is willing to accede to the patient's wishes (p. 141). The courts have also stated clearly that, when treatment has been limited in response to a request from a patient or his surrogate, neither the physician nor the institution is at risk of criminal or civil liability for the subsequent death of the patient. In spite of this, physicians and hospital attorneys have frequently continued to express unjustified fears about the risks of litigation and, for this reason, many continue to seek prior court approval for withdrawal of treatment, particularly of ANH.

Whilst the issue of autonomy is relatively straightforward when the patient is competent, the vegetative patient presents a more difficult problem. There is a natural wish to ensure that the incompetent patient should be protected from treatment that would likely be refused if that were possible. The problem is how to respect autonomy by discovering what the patient would likely want in the present circumstances. The American courts have identified two means of identifying this.

The first, the **subjective standard**, is the most satisfactory but is unfortunately the least often available. This is when the patient has previously expressed a treatment preference. Evidence for the patient's wishes may range from a written living will to remembered casual conversations. There is much legal debate about how clear and convincing this evidence should be before it is acted on. A written statement will always be regarded as more reliable evidence of the settled will of the patient but courts have often been willing to take note of the reported views of the patient. Such reports depend on the statements of family members, acting as witnesses or surrogates, and this may raise the issue of their statements being influenced by the personal views of these reporters. Therefore, when more than one witness can testify to the patient's views the court is more likely to take notice of these. Even when there is a written statement, whether or not as a formal living will, there is often the problem of whether it is sufficiently specific. Only occasionally will it actually request no tube feeding if permanently vegetative. More often it expresses only a general wish for no heroic or artificial means of life support if terminally ill, or if no longer able to communicate clearly, or to look after their personal needs. There is also the debate about how valid is a living will that was enacted years previously when the person was in good health. Some argue that people might change their minds in the present circumstances (p. 80). This seems unlikely to apply to the vegetative patient who is unaware of his condition, as distinct from a conscious patient who is now severely ill or disabled.

The *Cruzan* case that reached the US Supreme Court (p. 198) turned on the stance of the State of Missouri that it would allow withdrawal of ANH only if there was clear and convincing evidence of the patient's own wishes (9). Although the Supreme Court upheld the right of Missouri to demand this standard of evidence it did not require other states to do so. Indeed, a dissenting judge asserted that requiring this evidentiary standard would severely limit the rights of incompetent patients to appropriate treatment, while a commentator described it as an impractical standard that few cases would ever satisfy. In practice, only the states of Missouri and New York, and possibly Maine, employ such a rigid doctrine (10).

When no clear statement of the patient's wishes is available, the surrogate decision makers can have recourse to a **substituted judgment**. This entails trying to imagine what the patient would have wanted in the present circumstances. The surrogate is urged to have in mind the values and opinions of the patient, and also to take into account expressions of relevant treatment preferences by the patient that were not considered sufficiently secure on their own to form the basis for a subjective judgment. Studies comparing the views of competent patients and of their family members about what that patient would likely want in future circumstances, such as a wish for resuscitation, intensive care or rescue surgery, have shown a marked discrepancy between what patients wanted and what their family believed they would want. Although substituted judgment was favoured by the President's Commission (11) it has been criticized as more likely to reflect the values and biases of the surrogates than the views of the patient and several judges have called it 'a cruel charade'(12).

Best interests

When there is no evidence about the patient's preferences an **objective judgment** may be made on the basis of assessing the patient's best interests. It is almost certainly the most common means of deciding about limiting treatment, and one that conforms to the established ethical and medical principle of choosing the line of action most likely to ensure that the burdens of medical treatment do not outweigh the benefits. Although lack of benefit is the dominant factor in vegetative cases, there are some who hold that a decision to withdraw treatment based on best interests should require a clearer demonstration of undoubted burdens than if some evidence is available about the patient's wishes. That vegetative patients are unable to suffer has posed a problem for some when trying to identify burdens. Indeed, in the cases of *Conroy* and *Jobes* the New Jersey Supreme Court stipulated that only if continued treatment was going to inflict severe pain would withdrawal be justified (13). Others have, however, protested that this was to take too narrow a definition of burden (p. 193). Several courts have specifically rejected consideration of quality of life in assessing best interests, while accepting that they would respect the right of competent patients to refuse treatment either now or in a previous statement. Surely, most such patients are refusing treatment on the basis of the quality of life expected with that treatment? The problem that concerns some is judging the quality of someone else's life when that person cannot be consulted, as discussed in Chapter 8 (p. 104).

There remains, therefore, some room for debate as to how to determine the best interests of a vegetative patient, whom some have claimed can have no interests. The question of **who** should decide about the patient's best interests is discussed later (p. 134). One approach to best interests that avoids involving a decision maker who is asked to focus on this particular patient is to consider what most reasonable people would want if permanently vegetative. There is now good evidence, reviewed in Chapter 6, that most people do not regard continued survival as in the best interests of any permanently vegetative patient, and that many believe they would want treatment withdrawn if they themselves were in that state. Indeed, it has been asserted that the time has come to re-examine the presumption that treatment should be continued in order to prolong life, because this appears to be against the health goals of most citizens (14). It has even been suggested that there should be a 'vegetative state treatment statute' to mandate withdrawal unless the patient has previously expressed a contrary desire (15). Some who oppose such withdrawal refuse to accept that vegetative patients are a special case, and believe that they should be regarded simply as very severely disabled. They then cite the Americans with Disabilities Act of 1990 that makes it unlawful to discriminate against persons with disabilities, and pro-life groups have argued that this pro-hibits the withdrawal of life-sustaining treatment from vegetative patients. In fact, lawyers opposing treatment withdrawal in a vegetative case have not invoked this Act in court. However, in the case of the anencephalic *Baby K* a court maintained that the mother's wish for continued ventilation should be respected under this Act, although physicians had declared it to be futile treatment (16).

Right to privacy and to liberty

One or other or both of these constitutional rights have been relied on in many court decisions to abate treatment, from *Quinlan* to *Cruzan*. These are interpreted as the right to choose how to live one's life, free from the interference of the state. In the medical context this is taken to include the right to decide about how one is treated and in particular to be free of unwanted, burdensome or futile treatment. Although many state courts have regarded the right of privacy as a right to refuse treatment, in the early years some had been reluctant to extend this beyond reproductive decision making (6). The US Supreme Court in *Cruzan* based its support for the right to refuse unwanted treatment on the right of liberty rather than on the common law right of self-determination or the right of privacy (9). The right to freedom from cruel and unusual punishment has occasionally been claimed in courts as yet another reason for abating treatment, but this has been regarded as inappropriate. Yet one commentator referred to vegeta-tive patients as being the victims of the technologic imperative of phys-icians, and as prisoners of technology (17).

Is life expectancy relevant?

The question is whether withdrawing treatment from a vegetative patient can be regarded as a natural extension of the practice accepted for other types of patient, many of whom are terminally ill. In its 1982 statement, the AMA added that when a **terminally ill** patient's coma was beyond doubt irreversible, then all means of life support may be discontinued (irreversible coma was taken to include the vegetative state). In an expanded version of this statement in 1986, the reference to irreversible coma was qualified by 'even if death is not imminent' (18). This addendum was considered necessary because several statements about treatment withdrawal had referred to terminal illness and, as vegetative patients may live for years, it was difficult to claim that they were terminally ill. The President's Commission had cautioned against strict definitions of terminally ill or of when death should be considered imminent (11). Certainly, the courts have allowed a number of treatment withdrawals from competent patients who were not terminally ill (6,12). However, some courts have sought to limit decisions to withdraw treatment from incompetent patients to those who were terminally ill (often defined as an expectation of one year or less), unless there was good evidence of the patient's preference. Several living will statutes were originally limited to the terminally ill but since *Cruzan* most have been modified to include permanently vegetative patients. Whilst some courts have expanded the concept of terminally ill to include those with no hope of recovery, others have specifically stated that expectancy of life is not relevant for decisions about vegetative patients (12,19).

Who decides?

Whilst there is little debate about the dominance of the patient's wishes over all others in authorizing the doctor to act, there has been the debate described above about how clearly the patient's views have to have been expressed before being accepted. Absent such an acceptable declaration, the question is whether the *Quinlan* decision to leave it to the family and physicians, perhaps with the support of a hospital ethics committee, is acceptable, or whether and when judicial review is necessary.

Role of the courts

The year after *Quinlan,* the Massachussetts Supreme Court heard the *Saikewicz* case about withholding chemotherapy for leukaemia from a 67-year-old who had been mentally retarded all his life. This judge declared that the awesome question of either continuing or withholding potentially life-prolonging treatment was one for the courts of law and could not be granted to any other group (20). This provoked comments in the *New England Journal of Medicine* from its editor and from a law professor, who expressed astonishment and disbelief respectively at such a vote of no confidence in the ability of physicians and families to act in the best interests of an incapable patient (20,21). They noted that this went against both the *Quinlan* judgement and the medical policies for limiting treatment for the hopelessly ill that had been set out previously in the same journal (2,3,4).

In spite of this, the New York Appeal Court in 1980 in the case of *Fox,* an 83-year-old priest who was vegetative, declared that the neutral presence of the law was necessary to weigh the many factors relevant to a decision to disconnect life-support systems (22). This court acknowledged the concern expressed after the Massachusetts case but denied any mistrust of the judgement of physicians and families. 'Rather our decision recognizes that the societal interests to be safeguarded are so great that the courts have no choice but to intervene on a patient-to-patient basis'. After so many judgements approving treatment withdrawal in vegetative cases, many American courts have now explicitly stated that judicial review is usually unnecessary. It may, however, still be needed if a patient has no family or other surrogates, if there is reason to suspect the motives of the family, or if there is some dispute between the parties (6,12,23). The court's role would then normally be limited to the appointment of a *guardian ad litem* to act as surrogate. Not only are courts unnecessary but they are not well placed to make such decisions (24,25). They are slow and cumbersome and indeed several patients have died before their legal case was decided, but a later judgement was, none the less, given because the issue was regarded as important for future patients. As well as the delay, the expense and publicity are a deterrent, whilst in the words of one judge 'our legal system cannot replace the more intimate struggle that must be borne by the patient, those caring for the patient and those who care about the patient' (26).

Role of physicians

Some commentators have emphasized that, whatever medical expertise physicians may have in regard to the diagnosis and prognosis of such patients, they are no better placed than others to make ethical decisions about treatment withdrawal. This reaction against medical paternalism usually seeks to replace the physician as decision maker by the patient and family rather than by a court of law. However, in the early days of their involvement with these cases some lawyers stressed that the involvement of the courts was as much to protect physicians from the possible legal repercussions of their proposed actions as to safeguard patients. It was supposed (often rightly) that physicians feared being accused of assisting suicide or of practising euthanasia or even of committing homicide – fears that lawyers insisted were exaggerated, if not illusory. The only prosecution against a physician for withdrawing treatment was the *Barber* case in California in 1983 (p. 190). In dismissing the murder charge against two physicians, the Superior Court stated that a physician acting in 'good faith and within established professional standards' could not incur civil or criminal liability (6). Many other courts have subsequently accepted this principle when considering liability.

The contribution of physicians to decisions about the treatment of incompetent hopelessly ill patients was ignored in the *Cruzan* judgement (9). This was criticized on the grounds that physicians were likely often to have had views expressed to them by their patients as to how they would want to be treated, and they might therefore know more about their preferences than did some families (23,24,25). In the light of the *Cruzan* (p. 198) and *O'Connor* (p. 196) court cases (27), and of the subsequent Patient Self-Determination Act (28) discussed below, these commentaries have stressed the importance of doctors now seeking to initiate discussions with patients that will encourage them to make advance directives. If patients do not wish to do so formally in a directive, physicians should record whatever views have been expressed to them as useful evidence if and when the patient should become incompetent. Many declarations in courts and elsewhere have recommended that decisions should be made by the patient, family and physicians in collaboration. However, some have sought to limit the physician's role to determining the prognosis and informing the patient and/or the family of this, pointing out that a doctor has no special status for making moral decisions about whether or not treatment should be continued. This may seem out of touch with medical reality because physicians are frequently making such decisions (about terminally ill or moribund patients) without undue formality, and discussing the ethics of such decision making in their journals. In the case of vegetative patients, however, it seems reasonable to require, as some courts have recommended, that more than one doctor should give an opinion about the diagnosis and prognosis. There should be adequate professional consultation between physicians before agreeing to withdraw treatment, and these steps should all be documented. In *Quinlan*, the use of a hospital ethics committee was suggested, and in the *Conroy* case (a nonvegetative patient in a nursing home), reference to the Ombudsman for the Institutionalized Elderly was recommended – a provision that was available for such patients in the state of New Jersey (p. 193).

Role of families

Most courts have accepted that families and other close associates make the most suitable surrogate decision makers, on the assumption that they are likely to be best informed about the values of the patient and about any informal expressions of preference previously made by the patient. Apart from the early *Saikewicz* and *Fox* courts which recommended judicial review as a rule – judgements that did not in fact lead to such practice – the more recent *O'Connor* and *Cruzan* cases are the only ones that have specifically challenged the wisdom of relying on the family (27). In *O'Connor*, the New York Appeal Court disputed the wishes of her daughters to discontinue treatment because it doubted the validity of their mother's previously expressed wishes as reported by them, and it did not offer the family the alternative of a substituted or objective judgment (p. 196). In *Cruzan*, the Missouri Supreme Court claimed that her parents' assertion that she had stated that she would not wish to continue to live like this was not sufficiently clear and convincing evidence of her wishes to justify treatment withdrawal (p. 131). A public survey before the Supreme Court decision on *Cruzan* found that 88% favoured the family, 8% the physicians and 1% the court as the decision maker for treatment withdrawal (29). In the event, the US Supreme Court in 1990 supported the right of Missouri to deny the Cruzan family the right to make a decision, unless the patient's own wishes had been expressed in clear and convincing terms. Whilst not questioning the motives of the Cruzan family, the

Supreme Court went on to generalize about families (p. 198). They might, the majority judgement stated, 'have a strong feeling – not at all ignoble or unworthy, but not entirely disinterested either – that they do not wish to witness the continuation of a life which they regard as hopeless, meaningless and even degrading. But there was no automatic assurance that the views of those family members would necessarily be the same as the patient's would have been' (9,24). Dissenting justices maintained that the state's main purpose in such cases should be to determine the patient's wishes, and that the majority ruling limited the possibility of achieving that purpose because it deprived incompetent patients of those proxies best placed to speak for them. However, one of the concurring justices strongly supported advance directives and maintained that the constitution might require states to respect the decisions of duly appointed surrogates. Subsequent comment has emphasized that, although this ruling might increase legal uncertainty about family decision making, it was permissive only to Missouri and that no other states needed to accept it (23,24,30). In the several states that had already accepted family decisions there was no need to change practice. In fact, there have been few cases through the courts since *Cruzan* and it seems that the practices already evolved in the years before that case have simply continued, with families contributing largely to decision making, often based on best interests without an insistence on clear evidence of the patient's wishes.

Advance directives and appointing proxies

In view of the debate about the validity of proxy decision making as reliably reflecting the patient's likely wishes (31,32), an immediate consequence of the *Cruzan* decision was to boost the movement to encourage patients to make advance directives. The Federal Patient Self-Determination Act of 1990 aimed to do this (28). It required hospitals and nursing homes to advise patients on admission of their right to refuse treatment, and to make a directive or appoint a proxy to deal with future decision making if and when they were to become incompetent.

Living wills were introduced by a Chicago lawyer in 1969 (33) and, following *Quinlan*, were legalized in California's Natural Death Act in 1976. Largely in response to *Cruzan*, every state now has a statute for either a living will or a power of attorney for health, often both. These require professionals to follow a patient's advance directive or the decision of a person with power of attorney and they provide these professionals and their institutions with legal immunity from the consequences of complying with such treatment refusals. It has been emphasized that a living will need not have been written by a lawyer and should not need a lawyer to interpret it. In spite of this, only a small minority of people are supposed to have made such a will. Moreover, many wills are written in such general terms that it has been easy for reluctant physicians (and lawyers) to avoid complying with them, on the grounds that the condition that has eventuated or the treatment to be limited were not specifically covered in the wording of the will (34,35). Limitations on the use of such wills for vegetative patients were that many early statutes approved their application only for terminally ill patients and were sometimes limited to withdrawal only of extraordinary treatments, which was taken to exclude the withdrawal of ANH. Since the *Cruzan* case, many states have amended their statutes specifically to allow withdrawal of ANH from permanently vegetative patients. Even so, patients are now encouraged to state in their living will, if this is their wish, specific directions about ANH if they were to become vegetative, in addition to the generality of not wanting heroic measures if they were to become hopelessly or terminally ill. The ethical doubts about the validity of declarations made by healthy people about imagined later illness and incompetence have already been discussed (p. 131).

Because of the difficulty of living wills being made sufficiently specific to ensure that a patient's wishes are respected, it is considered much more protective of autonomy for a proxy decision maker to be appointed, whom the physicians can then consult. Whilst courts have been prepared to accept next of kin as proxies on an informal basis, the advantage of a designated proxy is that if there is disagreement among family members this authorizes one of them to speak for the patient. It also allows a patient to appoint someone other than their next of kin, such as a close friend or de facto partner, who is more aware of their currrent values. When encouraging patients to appoint proxies, physicians should encourage them to discuss their future wishes with these proxies. Unless this has been done, there is concern about whether proxy decision making will always reflect the patient's views or best interests (31,32,34,35).

Cause of death from a legal standpoint

Some have maintained, that as withdrawal of feeding so inevitably leads to death, it is an action intended to cause the patient's death that therefore constitutes homicide (or, if requested by a patient, suicide). This has led to supposed conflicts between the criminal and the civil law and to much debate about the distinction between killing and letting die (p. 113). The courts have consistently rejected these arguments, making it clear that the cause of death in such cases was the underlying disease that would long ago have caused the patient's death had there not been life-sustaining treatment. Stopping a treatment that has failed to benefit the patient even after a prolonged trial therefore lets the patient die rather than killing him. Some have sought to distinguish between an act and an omission, suggesting that there might be a difference between pulling up the tube (an act) and failing to connect the next bottle of fluid (an omission). However, like the distinction between withholding and withdrawing, the courts have rejected this distinction. As for the argument that the physician's legal duty to care for a patient always includes feeding, this has been rejected on the grounds that this is treatment and that there has never been a duty to provide treatment that brings no benefit. However, a clear distinction is seen between such withdrawal and a direct intervention to hasten death, such as a lethal injection. This would amount to active euthanasia, which is not legally tolerated in the US. Some opponents of withdrawing tube feeding from vegetative patients appear to base their objection on concern that this might be interpreted as sanctioning active euthanasia, an argument specifically rejected by the courts.

The only time that a doctor has been accused of murder for withdrawing tube feeding was in the *Barber* case in California, and the Superior Court in 1983 dismissed this indictment before the case came to trial (p. 190). That decision made clear that withdrawing any treatment considered not of benefit to the patient was acceptable medical practice and did not require prior judicial approval.

Refusal of institutions to withdraw or continue treatment

The courts have recognized that there are institutions that have been unwilling to withdraw treatment even when it has been ordered by a court.

Usually this has been because the institution had a mission statement (either explicit or implied by its affiliation, for example with the Catholic Church), but it may sometimes have been in support of individual physicians or nurses who had profound personal moral objections. It is accepted that some institutions have a right to pursue a sectarian philosophy of treatment, but this does not extend to public hospitals. It is easy to say that any restrictions on possible treatment preferences should have been available to patients on admission, but this is unrealistic in the circumstances of patients who sustain acute brain damage and are rushed to the nearest acute hospital, or are subsequently transferred to the first long-term facility willing to accept them. While courts have usually dealt with the problem of unwillingness to comply by recommending transfer to a willing physician or institution, such transfer is not always possible. In three cases (*Requena*, *Jobes* and *Gray*) the courts ordered institutions that had objected, and had been unable to arrange transfer, to accede to these patients' requests to withdraw treatment (36).

Nursing homes, irrespective of any religious affiliation, are frequently unwilling to consider withdrawal of ANH for a number of reasons (37). They have fewer doctors, lawyers and ethics committees than acute hospitals and may be ignorant of the consensus about withdrawal that has emerged in recent years. They are also subject to Federal and State regulations devised to prevent abuse that do not apply to acute hospitals. These usually include a stipulation that every patient must be given adequate nutrition and hydration, and periodic surveys to check on compliance may require forms to be filled in for selected patients which ask if they are being adequately fed. There is no doubt that exceptions could be made for vegetative patients whose families wished to withdraw ANH but the nursing-home authorities are apt to interpret these regulations rigidly, from fear of overzealous officials enforcing them and of bad publicity. Indeed, families who request withdrawal are said to be likely to have this refused, and may even be threatened with being reported for abuse or asked to remove their vegetative relative (37).

Between 1984 and 1989, there were three court cases brought against institutions for having continued to treat vegetative patients against the wishes of the family (6). In two, the courts supported the withholding of payments from the institutions involved for treatment and care after it had been refused. In a plea after *Cruzan* for more precisely worded advance directives, it was suggested that if providers failed to heed such specific wishes then further reimbursement for care should be terminated (38).

A more vexed issue is whether patients have a legal right to demand the continuation of treatment that has been deemed nonbeneficial by physicians and by common consent. The ethical issues involved in such a situation have already been discussed (p. 106). The legal case that focused attention on this problem was that of *Helga Wanglie*. She was an 86-year-old who had been vegetative for about a year following an anoxic episode. For some 8 months the hospital had been advocating removal of the respirator but her husband (an attorney) and children refused. They maintained that the respirator was not ineffective because it was keeping her alive and that she would have wanted this (although initially having said that she had expressed no preferences). Both physicians and nurses were unwilling to continue what they regarded as inappropriate and nonbeneficial treatment. There was no financial interest in terminating treatment as the costs were covered by insurance. For 5 months the husband and his attorney searched unsuccessfully for another hospital to take her on transfer, but none would do so. Such refusals suggested that many professionals agreed that continued treatment was inappropriate. The hospital asked a court to appoint an independent conservator to decide about treatment, but the husband cross-filed to be appointed conservator. The court chose the husband who could therefore have his demand for continuing treatment respected, but the patient died 3 days later. This was after *Cruzan*, by which time many vegetative cases had come to court where the family's request for treatment refusal had been upheld. It seemed that the *Wanglie* court was unwilling to see a family's wishes frustrated, not only when refusing nonbeneficial treatment but also when they wanted it continued (39). A physician who was the ethics consultant from *Wanglie*'s hospital subsequently argued the opposing case (40).

The minimally conscious state

With the question of withdrawal of treatment from vegetative patients largely settled by reason of many court decisions, effectively endorsed by the Supreme Court opinions in *Cruzan*, a new area of uncertainty has emerged about the rights of persons in a minimally conscious state (MCS). The nature of this condition has already been described (p. 23). There have been two similar cases where courts have refused requests for treatment withdrawal from patients in this condition (41). Both were middle-aged men who had been in MCS for 11 and 4 years following head injuries. In each case, their wives related that their husbands had previously made comments about not being kept alive if hopelessly ill. In each case, the wives and children requested withdrawal but both patients had a mother and a sister who opposed this. In the case of *Martin*, the trial court agreed to withdrawal and the appeal court affirmed this, but in 1995 the Michigan Supreme Court reversed the decision (42). In the *Wenland* case, the Probate judge in 1998 claimed that California case law on persons in a vegetative state did not give adequate guidance to decide about this case, but he gave the wife authority to refuse all other treatments for her husband (43). The California court of appeal has still to give a final judgement on this case. Both courts considered that, for a nonvegetative patient, there had to be clear and convincing evidence of the patient's own wishes before ANH could be withdrawn. Both courts were fearful of a slippery slope to legalized euthanasia if either substituted judgment or best interests were the basis of a decision to withdraw treatment in such a case. The *Martin* court considered that his awareness, though limited, might allow him to be able to experience pain and to suffer distress from insight into his condition, but that this awareness might also allow him some enjoyment of his continued life. Rather than these being arguments in favour of continued treatment, some commentators (41) thought the opposite, and one observed that this court decision meant that the more the patient suffered the longer he was condemned to live (44).

Treatment withdrawal was also refused in Wisconsin for another MCS case (*Edna*), a 73-year-old woman with advanced Alzheimer's disease (45). Her sister recalled that, many years before this, the patient, a vibrant active journalist, had said that she would rather die of cancer than lose her mind. As her guardian, her sister requested cessation of feeding, and she was supported by several other relatives, the hospital ethics committee and her *guardian ad litem*. The circuit court decided that it did not have authority to grant the request as the patient was not in a vegetative state. The Supreme Court in 1997 agreed that a best interests judgment by a guardian was allowable only for vegetative patients. For other cases there had to be an advance directive or other clear statement of the patient's desires. As in the courts mentioned above, this court referred to fear of the slippery slope to legalized euthanasia if this line was not drawn. To insist on an advance directive that specifically referred to the MCS as distinct from the vegetative state is clearly unrealistic.

A commentary on this case drew attention to several previous court decisions that had specifically indicated that ANH could be withdrawn from nonvegetative patients (46). In the *Conroy* case, the New Jersey Supreme Court in 1985 explicitly stated that under the limited-objective test treatment could be withdrawn from nonvegetative patients (p. 192). There should, however, be **some** trustworthy evidence that the patient would have refused this treatment and it should be clear that the burdens of continued life outweighed the benefits. The Arizona Supreme Court in 1987, in deciding on a vegetative case (*Rasmussen*), did not limit best interests criteria for treatment withdrawal to vegetative patients (47). The Washington Supreme Court made a similar declaration about *Grant* in 1988 (48). More recently, since *Cruzan*, when the Supreme Court of Georgia in *Jane Doe* ruled that the right to refuse treatment is not lost because an incompetent has failed to leave a treatment directive and it expressly rejected arguments that the right to refuse treatment by surrogates acting in the patient's best interests should be limited to patients in a vegetative state (49). As medical knowledge about the diagnosis and prognosis of the minimally conscious state increases and becomes more widely known, it seems likely that the law may come to accept that it may be in the best interests of some such patients to have life-sustaining treatment withdrawn.

REFERENCES

1 *In re Quinlan.* 70.NJ 10 355 A2d 647 (1976)
2 Report of the Clinical Care Committee of the Massachusetts General Hospital. Optimum care for hopelessly ill patients. *N Engl J Med* 1976; 295: 362–4
3 Rabkin MT, Gillerman G, Rice JD. Orders not to resuscitate. *N Engl J Med* 1976; 295: 364–6
4 Bok S. Personal directions for care at the end of life. *N Engl J Med* 1976; 295: 367–9
5 Fried C. Terminating life support: out of the closet. *N Engl J Med* 1976; 295: 390–91
6 Weir RF, Gostin L. Decisions to abate life-sustaining treatment for non–autonomous patients. *JAMA* 1990; 264: 1846–53
7 Beresford HR. The Brophy case: whose life is it? *Neurology* 1981; 37: 1357–8
8 Justice Cardozo. In *Schloendorff* v. *Society of New York Hospitals.* (1914) 211 NY 125.105 NE 92–3
9 *Cruzan* v. *Director Missouri Department of Public Health.* 110 SCt 2841 (1990)
10 Bernat JL. *Ethical issues in neurology.* Boston: Butterworth-Heinemann, 1994
11 President's Commission for the Study of Ethical Problems in Medicine. *Deciding*

to Forego Life-Sustaining Treatment. Washington DC: US Govt. Printing Office, 1983

12 Emanuel EJ. A review of the ethical and legal aspects of terminating medical care. *Am J Med* 1988; 84: 291–300

13 Emanuel EJ. What criteria should guide decision makers for incompetent patients? *Lancet* 1988; 1, 170–71

14 Angell M. After Quinlan: the dilemma of the persistent vegetative state. *N Engl J Med* 1994; 330: 1524–5

15 Shapiro RS. The case of LW: an argument for a permanent vegetative state statute *Ohio State Law J* 1990; 51: 439

16 Schrode KE. Life in limbo: revising policies for permanently unconscious patients. *Houston Law Rev* 1995; 31: 1609–68

17 Angell M. Prisoners of technology: the case of Nancy Cruzan. *N Engl J Med* 1990; 322: 1226–8

18 American Medical Association Council on Ethical and Judicial Affairs. Withholding and withdrawing life prolonging medical treatment. *JAMA* 1986; 256: 471

19 Emanuel EJ. Should physicians withhold life-sustaining care from patients who are not terminally ill? *Lancet* 1988; 1; 106–8

20 Curran WJ. The Saikewicz decision. *N Engl J Med* 1978; 298: 499–500

21 Relman AS. The Saikewicz decision: Judges as physicians. *N Engl J Med* 1978; 298: 508–9

22 McCormick RA. The Fox case. *JAMA* 1980; 244: 2165–66

23 Lo B, Steinbrook R. Beyond the Cruzan case: the US Supreme Court and medical practice. *Ann Intern Med* 1991; 114: 895–901

24 Annas GJ. Nancy Cruzan and the right to die. *N Engl J Med* 1990; 323: 670–73

25 Lo B, Rouse F, Dornbrand L. Family decision-making on trial. Who decides for incompetent patients? *N Engl J Med* 1990; 322: 1228–32

26 *In re Jobes* 108 NJ 394 529 A2d 434 (1987)

27 Gasner MR. *Cruzan* v. *Harmon* and in the matter of *O'Connor: J Am Geriatr Soc* 1990; 38: 594–9

28 Wolf SM, Boyle P, Callahan D et al. Sources of concern about The Patient Self-Determination Act. *N Engl J Med* 1991; 325: 1666–70

29 Coyle M. How Americans view high court. *Natl Law J* 1990; 26 February: 36–7

30 Thirty four Bioethicists. Bioethicists' statement on the US Supreme Court's Cruzan decision. *N Engl J Med* 1990; 323: 686–7

31 Emanuel EJ, Emanuel LL. Proxy decision-making for incompetent patients; an ethical and empirical analysis. *JAMA* 1992; 267: 2067–71

32 Lynn J. Procedures for making medical decisions for incompetent adults. *JAMA* 1992; 267: 2101–4

33 Kutner L. Due process of euthanasia: the living will, a proposal. *Indiana Law J* 1969; 44: 539

34 Orentlicher D. The illusion of patient choice in end-of-life decisions. *JAMA* 1992; 267: 2101–4

35 Annas GJ. The health care proxy and the living will. *N Engl J Med* 1991; 324: 1210–13

36 Miles SH, Singer PA, Siegler M. Conflicts between patient's wishes to forgo treatment and the policies of health care facilities. *N Engl J Med* 1989; 321: 48–50

37 Meisel A. Barriers to forgoing nutrition and hydration in nursing homes. *Am J Law Med* 1995; 21: 335–82

38 Rie MA. Practicing medicine, fiduciary trust, privacy and public moral interloping after *Cruzan. J Med Philos* 1992; 17: 647–64

39 Angell M. The case of Helga Wanglie. *N Engl J Med* 1991; 325: 511–12

40 Miles SH. Informed demand for 'non-beneficial' medical treatment. *N Engl J Med* 1991; 325: 512–15

41 Nelson LJ, Cranford RE. Michael Martin and Robert Wenland: beyond the vegetative state. *J Contemp Health Law Policy* 1999; 15: 427–53

42 *In re Martin,* N.W. 2d 399 (Mich. 1995), cert. denied, 516 U.S. 113 (1996)

43 *In re Conservatorship of Wenland* Cal Sup Ct (1997, 1998)

44 Cranford RE. The more you suffer, the longer you live. *Bioeth Exam* 1999; 2: 1–2

45 *In re Edna MF,* 563 N.W. 2d 485 (Wisc 1997) cert. denied

46 Shapiro RS. In re Edna MF: case law confusion in surrogate decision making. *Theor Med* 1999; 20: 45–54

47 *Rasmussen* v. *Fleming,* 154 Ariz. 207, 741 P.2d 674 (1987)

48 *In re Grant,* 109 Wash. 2d 545, 747 P.2d 445 (1987), modified 757 P.2d 534 (1988)

49 *In re Jane Doe,* 262 Ga. 389,418 S.E.2d 3 (1992)

10

Legal issues in Britain

The medical profession in Britain was reluctant during the 1970s and 1980s to adopt formal approaches to decisions to limit treatment. Persisting with nonbeneficial treatment in various clinical situations was seen as largely an American problem, in spite of clear evidence that it also occurred in Britain. As for the legality of this problem, the eminent physician who drew attention to this contrast with America added that in Britain 'the medical team is under few constraints – familial, medical and, least of all, legal – to act as it sees fit in the best interest of the patient' (1). Eventually a single case was to change all that. In April 1989, the teenager *Anthony Bland* suffered anoxic brain damage when crushed in a football stadium. After 4 months in a vegetative state, his parents requested withdrawal of tube feeding and his physician, who was in agreement, sought the advice of the local coroner. His view was that if *Bland* then died he would have no option as Coroner but to recommend criminal proceedings and he advised seeking further legal advice. It was to be more than 3 years later (and 16 years after *Quinlan*) before that case reached the highest courts in the land, which then established the conditions required for withdrawal of ANH from vegetative patients to be legally acceptable in the future (p. 207).

In 1990 there was a brief news item in the *Lancet* reporting the *Cruzan* case with a more extended report by an American in that journal's 'Medicine and the Law' section in January 1991 (2). In that same issue, an Institute of Medical Ethics report concluded that it was morally justified to withdraw ANH from vegetative patients (3). It acknowledged, however, that even if such a decision were made with the full support of the doctors and the family the legal position in the UK was unclear, and it urged professional bodies to make recommendations about the appropriateness of such a decision. A few months later, the author of this book, who had been associated with the above report, wrote with a solicitor an article in the *British Medical Journal* that contrasted the busy legal scene in the US with the legal vacuum in Britain (4). They pointed out that in Britain there were no constitutional rights to privacy and liberty and no legislation to underpin the use of living wills, although it had been recognized that English law already required doctors to act according to a patient's previously expressed wishes (5). They also emphasized that family members in Britain had no legal right to make treatment decisions for incompetent adults (6). Only doctors could make such decisions, based on the best interests of their patients, albeit after due consultation with families. These authors noted that on the few occasions when the British courts had considered decisions about the medical treatment of incompetent patients they had preferred a best interests approach rather than the substituted judgment frequently relied on in American courts.

However, in the specific case of withdrawing ANH from a vegetative patient they considered it uncertain whether British courts would follow the American precedent of rejecting an allegation of homicide. They then compared the coroner's advice in the *Bland* case with a similar case in Scotland where the central legal office for the Scottish health boards had given different advice. This was that the procurator fiscal service (which investigates suspected crimes in Scotland) would not consider such a medical decision inappropriate. It advised securing a second medical opinion and **consulting** the relatives, but not asking for their **consent** because, as in England, relatives in Scotland have no legal right to consent to or refuse treatment on behalf of an incompetent adult. Treatment withdrawal proceeded in the Scottish case and this was reported in a TV documentary and also in the print press where a Home Office spokesman said 'The law in England is quite specific. We are talking about murder and we don't believe any changes would be proper' (7). Yet another TV documentary drew attention to the dilemma of the *Bland* family, seemingly prevented by law from doing their best for their son. This came to the attention of the Member of Parliament who was chairman of the Select (Parliamentary) Committee on the Health Service who took the matter up with the Minister for Health. Her response was that this matter was nothing to do with the Department of Health but one related to the criminal law.

Meanwhile, lawyers for the hospital trust caring for *Bland* had decided to take the case to the Family Division of the High Court in London that deals with the welfare of minors and incompetent adults. Aware of the controversy about the *Bland* case, the Medical Ethics Committee of the BMA produced, in September 1992, a discussion paper on the treatment of patients in the vegetative state (8). This cited many references to American cases and to the recent papers in the British medical literature mentioned above. It referred to a previous statement in the BMA Euthanasia Report (p. 116) in support of its conclusion that ANH was medical treatment that could reasonably be withdrawn from a permanently vegetative patient. It recommended that, before doing so, two additional independent medical opinions be sought. It recommended that withdrawal should not be considered until a patient had been vegetative for a year (this was 2 years before the US Task Force reported prognostic data for the first time). Although only a discussion paper which was later modified, the *Bland* courts relied heavily on this document as evidence that withdrawal of ANH was 'in accord with a responsible body of medical opinion'. This was a phrase commonly referred to in English civil courts when deciding that a given treatment had not been negligent, since the *Bolam* case in 1957 (9).

The *Bland* case in the courts

In November 1992 the President of the Family Division in the High Court heard the *Bland* case. Since the Mental Health Act of 1959, English law no longer grants a *parens patriae* role to courts when deciding about treatment for incompetent adults, although this still applies for patients who are wards of court. The Hospital Trust could therefore seek only a declaration that it would not be unlawful to withdraw ANH. This was opposed by the Official Solicitor in his traditional role as *guardian ad litem* for an incompetent patient. Because of the significance of this case for public policy the court invited the Attorney General to brief counsel to appear as *amicus curiae*. The medical witnesses agreed that *Bland* was in a permanent vegetative state, and that continuing treatment was not in *Bland*'s best interests, although one held that ANH was not medical treatment and therefore should not be withdrawn. His father gave evidence that he was sure that his son would not wish to go on living like this – but there was no suggestion that he had ever expressed such a view himself.

Counsel for the Trust maintained that an incompetent patient should not be disadvantaged in comparison to one who was competent and who would probably refuse such treatment and that doctors and nurses should not be at risk of legal repercussions if they acted in what they regarded as their patient's best interests, and in accord with good medical practice. He noted that the English courts had recently allowed doctors not to intervene to save the lives of badly handicapped infants who were not terminally ill because of the anticipated quality of life if they were to survive (10,11).

For the Official Solicitor, counsel argued that ANH was basic care and not medical treatment. He dismissed the reference to previous infant cases where pain and suffering were reasons to limit treatment as irrelevant because all the experts had agreed that *Bland* could not experience pain and suffering. He argued that to stop feeding him would be like cutting the rope of a suspended climber, or the air supply of a diver – in fact, murder.

For the Attorney General, counsel considered it unhelpful to have an absolutist position on these matters. He maintained that there was a difference between allowing and causing death. He considered that to ignore the quality of life was to show lack of respect for the sanctity of life. He referred at length to the *Cruzan* case with extracts in particular from the dissenting opinions and these were quoted again in the judgement.

In that judgement, Sir Stephen Brown, the President of the Family Division, accepted that ANH was medical treatment and that the cause of death after its withdrawal would be the initial severe brain damage (12). He noted that four of the five testifying doctors agreed that withdrawal would be 'in accordance with good medical practice, as stated in the BMA document, and would also be in accordance with the true benefit to *Anthony Bland*'. Such a decision would accord with those taken in other common law jurisdictions. He therefore declared that the physicians could lawfully discontinue all life-sustaining treatment. As for future cases, he considered that although such a decision was one for medical practitioners, the approval of the court should be sought for each case as a safeguard and for the reassurance of the public. At least two responsible medical opinions should be available to the court. In spite of this last ruling, the interesting feature of this judgement was that it relied on doctors both to decide about the best interests of the patient and about the appropriateness of withdrawing ANH.

The Official Solicitor appealed and less than 3 weeks later three judges unanimously upheld the ruling of the lower court (12). The Official Solicitor appealed to the House of Lords where five law lords heard the case and unanimously dismissed the appeal in February 1993. This support for the original ruling by all eight judges in two appeal courts contrasts with the American appellate courts where most decisions about such cases have been by narrow majorities.

However, all eight judges wrote separate opinions on why they supported the original judgement, as set out elsewhere (p. 209). These revealed considerable differences in their views, although none declared dissent. All were agreed that sanctity of life was not an absolute principle, and that competent patients had a right to refuse treatment even if this resulted in earlier death than would be expected with that treatment. Seven mentioned euthanasia, to dismiss it on the grounds that no external agency or act (such as a lethal injection) was involved in bringing about death. Six of the eight, agreed in various phrases, that there was no benefit to *Bland* in extending his life in this state. Some stated that it was in his best interests to have treatment discontinued (rather than to die), but others believed that he had no interests. Three judges referred to the courts in South Africa and New Zealand that had approved treatment withdrawal a few months before the first *Bland* court (pp. 204 and 206). In assessing the status of ANH as medical treatment two judges found it more easily described as a part of medical **care** – a more inclusive term for what doctors may or may not provide. Two judges were unhappy about relying either on the doctors involved in a case or on generally accepted medical opinion to decide either about a patient's best interests or that treatment should be withdrawn. In contrast, two considered that the role of the law was to provide protection for doctors taking legitimate but difficult decisions. Two expressed caution about allowing families to make these decisions. One pointed out that doctors can already proceed to treat incompetent patients in their best interests by the doctrine of necessity. That most often applied to saving life in emergencies but when an English court (in *Re F*) had declared the sterilization of a mentally handicapped adult to be lawful the judge pointed out that this extended the doctrine of necessity to a nonurgent, non-life-saving situation (6). Two judges stressed that their decision applied only to cases where the patient resembled *Bland* in being insensate; cases with slight awareness might be dealt with differently. One appeal court judge noted that the question of resource allocation could not be ignored, but felt that that was a matter for health authorities rather than the courts. Two made extensive reference to cases in other jurisdictions and one concluded that there was a community of view in the course of development and acceptance throughout the common law world on the legal aspects of discontinuing treatment.

Two regretted that English courts no longer had *parens patriae* powers to decide about treatment for incompetent adults, and could therefore only declare that a specific treatment was not unlawful. Three judges accepted that routine court referral should be only for the time being, one of whom hoped that it would soon be possible to relax this rule so that only cases with particular problems would then need to come to court. However, three of the law lords were strongly of the opinion that Parliament ought to consider legislation rather than leaving it to judges to do their best with existing law, where there was a conflict between civil and criminal liability. One law lord concluded that he felt profound misgivings about almost every aspect of this case, the resolution of which had called for 'distortion of a legal structure which is already morally and intellectually misshapen'.

Immediate reactions to the *Bland* decision

There was extensive coverage of each of these court hearings and press reaction was largely favourable. Doctors, on the whole, were satisfied with the outcome and an editorial in the *British Medical Journal* asserted that the decision brought Britain into line with other jurisdictions (13). There followed three letters of dissent. The medical witness who had opposed withdrawal of ANH in the court repeated his assertion that ANH was not medical treatment, and suggested that we should find better means of ending the lives of such patients (14). A doctor from 'Healthcare Opposed to Euthanasia' urged the profession, society and the law to think again (15). Another doctor wrote to clarify the Roman Catholic opposition (16), quoting a statement on behalf of the English and Welsh bishops (17). In spite of this, there were two contributions to the Catholic newspaper, *The Tablet*, affirming that the decision was compatible with Catholic tradition (18,19).

A legal commentator in the *Lancet* after the first court decision considered it gave little comfort to doctors who would have to face a traumatic court hearing every time they made a decision to withdraw ANH from a vegetative patient (20). It was, surely, she went on, the function of Parliament to extend the law to state clearly when an act of murder may be deemed lawful, rather than leaving this to a series of decisions by High Court judges. In this, she was anticipating the views later expressed by the law lords. Following the Court of Appeal decision another legal commentator in the *Lancet* considered it inappropriate to require every future case to come to court to allay public concern (21). That concern, she believed, would have been better directed at the delay in withdrawing treatment from *Bland*, who should have been allowed to die long ago when a simple statement by the Attorney General or the Director of Public Prosecution could have ended the fears of the doctors. In view of the fact that doctors were frequently making decisions about withholding or withdrawing treatment, it seemed to her unjustified to impose an artificial constraint for vegetative patients by requiring a court declaration. An anonymous editorial in the *Lancet* later observed that the ultimate decision in the House of Lords was suffused with uncertainty and, indeed, would probably not have been unanimous without the agreement to include the exhortation to Parliament to tidy up the law (22). It stated that doctors should not be expected to bring these tragedies to an end only by an act of murder, albeit made lawful by a court. It concluded that 'we fail to see why their lordships could not have pronounced more helpfully'.

House of Lords Select Committee on Medical Ethics

This was set up in response to the call for parliamentary involvement in the PVS issue, as well as concern about euthanasia raised by the *Cox* case that was in the High Court shortly before the *Bland* case (p. 116). One Lord unsuccessfully moved an amendment to have the committee's title changed to 'Euthanasia', an indication that a major focus of concern about the *Bland* decision was that it seemed to some that it sanctioned euthanasia. The committee was chaired by a neurologist and had a surgeon among its members. Between April and November 1993, it heard evidence from 20 individuals and received 69 written submissions amounting to 282 pages. Religious organizations accounted for 29% of submissions and of pages, with 35% of such submissions and 47% of pages coming from Roman Catholic organizations – reflecting the emphasis on euthanasia. The committee reported in February 1994 (23).

The report recommended no change in the law to permit euthanasia or physician-assisted suicide, and it was these conclusions that captured media attention. However, it strongly endorsed the right of a competent patient to refuse all medical treatment. For incompetent patients it recommended that a treatment-limiting decision should be taken jointly by all members of the health-care team, together with the family or close associates of the patient, on the grounds that further treatment would add nothing to the patient's well-being as a person. That decision should not be influenced by the availability of resources. It favoured the development of advance directives but considered specific legislation unnecessary. It did not favour the more widespread development of proxy decision making, as proxies might have mixed motives when making such a decision.

Regarding permanently vegetative patients, it recommended that the colleges and faculties of all health professions should develop diagnostic criteria and a code of practice for management. The 1996 report of the Royal College of Physicians on the permanent vegetative state (24) and the 1999 BMA guidance on limiting life-prolonging treatment (25) could be regarded as responses to this. The Select Committee supported the proposal in a recent Law Commission consultation paper (26) to set up a new judicial forum to authorize the initiation, withholding or withdrawal of treatment considered in a patient's best interests, where such approval was thought necessary. It supported the Law Commission's proposal that such approval should always be required for procedures in a special category (which would include withdrawal of ANH). Thus far, the committee had done little to alter the post-*Bland* status quo.

However, it then went on to report that it had been unable to reach a conclusion on whether or not to regard ANH as medical treatment – making it unique among all previous official bodies, such as medical associations and courts of law, that had pronounced on this matter. It went on to state, however, that 'the question [of its withdrawal] need not, indeed should not, usually be asked'. This was because the committee concluded that if antibiotics had been withheld earlier *Bland* would have succumbed much sooner to the inevitable complication of infection. Therefore, it concluded that it should never be necessary to consider withdrawal of nutrition and hydration, except when it was evidently burdensome. That conclusion was against all the medical evidence that had recorded the survival of many vegetative patients for years after a decision to withhold all treatment for complications – the very reason why the issue of withdrawal of ANH had arisen. By deciding that there was no problem the committee was able to ignore the pleas from the *Bland* judges to consider legislation to clarify the issue for doctors and lawyers. It is believed that these unhelpful conclusions were agreed as the price of producing a unanimous report. That several cases have continued to come to court every year over the 10 years since *Bland* indicates that it was unreasonable to declare that there was no medical or legal problem awaiting a solution.

Practice Notes of the Official Solicitor

A month after the Select Committee reported, the Official Solicitor to the Supreme Court issued a Practice Note on the vegetative state (27). This stated that the prior sanction of a High Court judge would be required in virtually all cases before termination of ANH for patients in a vegetative state (in England and Wales). An application would need to be made to the Family Division of the High Court with medical reports from the treating doctor and from an independent second practitioner indicating that the patient had been in a vegetative state for at least a year, as required by the BMA guidelines. The applicant could be the next of kin of the patient or the relevant health authority, which in any event ought to be a party. The Official Solicitor, who would act as *guardian ad litem* and brief counsel to appear on behalf of the patient, would commission a further independent medical report. The case would normally be heard in chambers with the judgement given in open court. The relief sought would be a declaration by the court that the plaintiffs and/or the responsible medical practitioners may lawfully discontinue all life-sustaining treatment (including ventilation, nutrition and hydration by artificial means) designed to keep X alive in his existing persistent vegetative state, and that they need not furnish medical treatment except for the sole purpose of enabling X to end his life and to die peacefully with the greatest dignity and the least distress. The patient's previously expressed views, either in writing or otherwise, would be a very important component in the decisions of the doctors and the court.

This was replaced by an expanded version in 1996 (28), which took account of several court judgements since *Bland.* It now stated that the diagnosis should be made in accordance with up-to-date medical guidelines, and reference was made to the 1996 Royal College of Physicians' report (24). Following this report's recommendation, it was accepted that for nontraumatic cases applications could be made after only 6 months in the vegetative state. From this report it also adopted the advice that the experts providing second opinions should ask medical and other clinical staff and relatives about the reactions and responses of the patient. However, it noted that the views of the next of kin or other close associates could not act as a veto to an application, although the court should take them into account. The important role of the medical opinion was to ensure that the patient was not sentient. Cases would normally be heard in open court but with steps taken to preserve the anonymity of the patient and the family, as well as the involved hospital or Trust. The order restricting publicity would continue to have effect after the death of the patient. It noted that a representative of the Official Solicitor would normally interview the next of kin and others close to the patient as well as seeing the patients and his carers.

Law Commission recommendations

The 1993 consultation paper from this body was available to the Select Committee and it led to a final report, *Mental incapacity*, in 1995 (29), which made frequent reference back to the report of the Select Committee. It responded to that committee's request for a specific definition of what factors would be relevant in determining 'best interests'. It noted that there had been vehement criticism of the assumption that, if a doctor acted in accordance with a body of medical opinion, he or she not only would not be negligent but could be regarded as having acted in the best interests of an incompetent patient. In assessing the best interest of PVS patients, the Commission considered that regard should be had to the ascertainable past and present wishes and feelings of these persons and the factors that they would consider if able to do so, taking account of the views of other people whom it was appropriate and practicable to consult about these factors. In regard to advance directives, it recommended that these should not be limited to terminal conditions, nor should they exclude refusal of life-sustaining treatments. An advance refusal should not preclude basic care (maintaining bodily cleanliness, alleviating severe pain and providing **direct** oral nutrition and hydration). Direct here appeared to mean in contrast to artificial or tube feeding.

The Commission, from its consultations, was not persuaded that decisions about withdrawing ANH could always be avoided, as the Select Committee had asserted. Such withdrawals should be declared lawful provided that certain statutory requirements were met. This would apply to a patient who was unconscious, had no activity in the cerebral cortex and had no prospect of recovery. The reference to no cortical activity was unfortunate in the light of recent medical evidence of residual activity in this part of the brain in some vegetative patients (p. 17), and the willingness of courts to allow withdrawal of ANH in spite of some evidence of cortical activity (p. 162). The term persistent vegetative state was purposefully avoided, according to the report, lest doctors who had not made this specific diagnosis might not see any need to seek legal approval for withdrawal. Unless there was a valid advance directive, the withdrawal of ANH would require either approval of the (newly proposed) Court of Protection, the consent of an attorney or court appointed manager or, if the Secretary of State decided so to provide, a certificate by an independent medical practitioner. This last was the device proposed to avoid the need to continue taking all cases to court. Such practitioners would be appointed for this purpose, and the order to allow this should be approved by each House of Parliament.

Some months after this the Scottish Law Commission published its *Report on incapable adults* (30), following an earlier discussion paper. It concluded that there should be new statutory provisions stating that it would be lawful to withhold or withdraw treatment that in the reasonable opinion of the doctors concerned would be unlikely to benefit the patient. The Commission decided against the restrictions on such decisions that the English Law Commission had proposed, and instead recommended that only in difficult and exceptional circumstances should the Court of Session be asked for a declarator that withdrawal would not be unlawful.

These proposals from the Select Committee and the Law Commissions have not so far been taken up by Parliament. However, following a consultation paper about the English Law Commission report, the Government issued a set of proposals (31). These accepted that there should be statutory guidance on how to determine the best interests of an incompetent person. There would be a new court to deal with making decisions on behalf of a person without capacity (an apparent restoration of *parens patriae* powers). These proposals stated that serious health-care decisions such as withdrawal of ANH from a patient in PVS, should remain a matter for this court and not be delegated to a court-appointed manager.

Further court cases

In the 7 years following the final *Bland* decision, 25 more similar cases were heard in the Family Division of the High Court, at a fairly steady rate of three or four each year. A senior lawyer from the Official Solicitor's department briefly reported the first ten cases in 1996 (32). In some cases, judges further developed the law in small ways and the more important of these cases will now be described.

The first to come to court after *Bland* was the *Frenchay* case – which is the name of the Trust, not the patient (33). This occurred in January 1994, before the publication of the Select Committee report or the Official Solicitor's Practice Note. It was unusual in several respects and was the only case since *Bland* that was taken to appeal. The conduct of this case attracted subsequent criticism from some legal commentators (34). *S* was a man of 24 who had been vegetative for more than 2 years following an anoxic episode. After 2 years, steps were begun to obtain legal permission to withdraw ANH but no application had been made when, 6 months later, his gastrostomy tube became blocked. His treating consultant took the view that as he had been vegetative for so long, and treatment withdrawal had already been discussed, it would not be in the patient's best interest to replace the tube. An urgent application for a declaration was made and a High Court judge heard the case the next day. The consultant told the court that he had support for his position from repeated discussions with other doctors over the last 2 years. A professor of neurology in 1992 had declared that there was no prospect of further recovery and he had more recently confirmed this opinion, although noting that the patient was very restless. A consultant neuropsychiatrist, who had seen him a year previously and saw him again after the tube blocked, had declared him to be in a vegetative state with no prospect of recovery. The patient had been in a specialist neurorehabilitation unit in October 1993 when the discharge note re-corded that he had many of the features of the persistent vegetative state. The nurses currently dealing with the patient supported the withdrawal of treatment as did his mother, who had long wanted him to be allowed to die. His father was more ambivalent and had indeed signed permission for replacement of the tube. Counsel appeared for the Official Solicitor, but with only 24 hours notice, he had been unable to secure an additional independent medical opinion. The judge granted the requested declaration but the Official Solicitor appealed and the next day the Court of Appeal unanimously upheld the initial judgement.

The grounds of appeal were that *S* and his *guardian ad litem* had been denied a fair and full opportunity to present all relevant material to the court; that the diagnosis of PVS could be questioned; and that too much attention had been paid by the judge to the doctor's assessment of the patient's best interests. Sir Thomas Bingham, the Master of the Rolls, who had previously heard the *Bland* appeal, considered that doctors in emergency situations might have to make decisions without referral to a court at all, or, if the case did come to court, it might not be possible to make presentations in the same leisurely way as in the *Bland* case. This did not justify reversing the judgement. As for the diagnosis it was accepted that the medical evidence was not as emphatic or unanimous as in the *Bland* case, but no doctor claimed that there was any cognitive function worth the name. As for the third point, they agreed that the court should reserve the ultimate power to review the doctor's decision – but considered that the judge who had heard the evidence had properly done this in the light of the House of Lords' judgements. This case showed how quickly the courts could respond to an emergency application – an answer to those who fear that routine court referral would make problems for doctors because of the slow process of the law. Since then, other cases of blocked feeding tubes have been dealt with at short notice by the courts.

Indeed, the next case was of this kind (35). *S* was a woman who had been vegetative for more than 2 years after neurosurgery for a brain tumour. She was cared for at home and when her tube blocked without warning her husband and children, who had strong religious faith, felt it was not right to replace the tube and prolong her life. The local NHS Trust made the application and although only notified late on a Friday afternoon the Official Solicitor managed to arrange an expert medical examination in time for the court hearing on the Saturday afternoon, when the necessary declaration was granted. The question of who should make the application and pay the costs for any future patients cared for at home was raised. The judge ruled that as the purpose of involving the court was to reassure the public, the party with the biggest purse should foot the bill – in effect the relevant health authority.

The next case, *Re G*, was a man of 28 who had had a severe head injury complicated by cardiac arrest, leaving him vegetative for more than 3 years. It was legally important in two respects. At a preliminary hearing, Sir Stephen Brown declared that such cases ought to be heard in open court to allow public debate about issues of such gravity (36). However, an order should be made to protect the privacy of the patient and family and, in order to preserve this, the name of the hospital, the Trust or the treating doctor should also not be identified. In the later case of *Re C* the question of press publicity was raised again and the President ruled that restrictions on identification were capable of enduring beyond the death of the patient (37). However, he later ruled that such orders to the press could not fetter the jurisdiction of a coroner to hold an inquest in open session. The other feature of *Re G* was that, although the patient's wife strongly supported the application to withdraw ANH, his mother opposed it. Her legal team had a report from a professor of neurology who, however, agreed with the other doctors about the diagnosis. The judge ruled that although the mother's views were relevant they could not act as a veto over the clear wishes of the wife and the opinion of the doctors and of the Official Solicitor (38).

There followed some unremarkable cases and then one that was unusual in two respects. One feature was that the patient had multiple injuries that resulted in his being ventilator-dependent and the family chose to withdraw ventilation rather than ANH. The other was that the family allowed him to be identified after the court case and his case was the subject of a television documentary in the series *The Decision*, which explored the feelings of people who had had to make critical decisions – in this case the parents.

At the end of 1995 and early in 1996 came two cases who died before reaching court – neither of them being cases of any urgency. There were also two cases in which procedures were begun but then abandoned. One was a young woman who was very severely brain damaged but known not to be vegetative, but where the mother maintained that her daughter had previously expressed a wish not be kept alive if in a severely brain damaged state. Although communication with this patient was very difficult, her mother and one doctor believed that she had indicated in her present state that she did not wish to kept alive. However, prolonged structured sessions with two different pairs of neuropsychologists revealed that she often indicated by nonverbal responses that she did wish to go on living (see p. 83). The application was immediately withdrawn. The other was a 6-week-old baby in which the difficulty at this age of making a firm diagnosis and prognosis led to the case being withdrawn. However, the following year the case of *Re C* (a baby in wardship) was completed in court (39). After meningitis in the first few weeks of life, this baby was left brain damaged and ventilator-dependent, and the court agreed to withdrawal of ventilation. This led to some discussion of whether withdrawal of ventilation needed a court order as is required for ANH (32). Ventilation did subsequently appear in the 1996 Practice Note as needing court approval.

In 1997–98 there were three cases in which the President granted declarations although the patients did not satisfy all the criteria laid down by the Royal College of Physicians. *Re D* concerned a 21-year-old woman who had suffered severe head injuries 8 years previously that left her with severe disabilities from permanent brain damage. She was at home with a full-time carer and very dissatisfied with her quality of life when she suffered a further brain insult that left her vegetative for the last 18 months. An application had already been made for a declaration to allow withdrawal of ANH when her feeding tube became detached and her treating physician and her mother were reluctant to replace it. The case came to court three days later (40). One independent expert witness for the Trust, a professor of neurology, said that many aspects of her responsiveness were in keeping with the vegetative state. However, she had a menace response, some primitive visual following, some nystagmoid responses of the eyes to caloric stimulation and some epileptic seizures. He did not believe that these meant any degree of awareness whatever, but because these aspects of the examination did not fulfil the 'other clinical features' part of the Royal College criteria it was difficult to diagnose her as in PVS by those criteria. He had sympathy for the application to withdraw ANH. A second independent witness for the Trust had no doubt that she was permanently vegetative regardless of not fulfilling certain features in the College criteria, which he considered a matter of some dispute among experts. Medical witness for the Official Solicitor accepted that when these eye signs were observed great caution had to be exercised in diagnosing the vegetative state. He believed, however, that *D* had no evidence of awareness and was therefore vegetative and that this state was permanent, but that because of the variation from the Royal College criteria he could not properly use the term PVS.

This was one of the few cases since *Bland* where counsel for the Official Solicitor opposed the granting of an application – on the grounds that the case breached the Royal College guidelines. However, he accepted that these were not statutory and therefore were open to interpretation by medical experts in any given case. The judge emphasized that all witnesses, including the patient's mother, held that the patient had no awareness of anything or anyone. Moreover, this patient satisfied all three of the primary criteria that the College report stated must all be fulfilled. It was only some of the 'other clinical features' of the report that she did not have. He therefore granted the declaration. Legal correspondents of both the *British Medical Journal* (41) and of the *Lancet* (42) commented on the case, the latter under the headline 'UK judge allows withdrawal of artificial feeding in prolonged non-PVS coma'. The medical aspects of these anomalies in the Royal College report have been discussed elsewhere (p. 14).

Re H was the second case with eye signs inconsistent with the 'other features' of the College criteria (43). This 24-year-old woman had been vegetative for more than 3 years since a severe head injury. The problem here was that there was some visual tracking and an occasional response to visual threat. An unusual number of experts gave evidence. No fewer than four consultant neurologists and a professor of neuropsychology examined the patient and the court also heard oral evidence from two nurses. All were agreed that there was no evidence of awareness and the neurologists considered her to be in PVS. The Official Solicitor did not oppose the application, which was granted.

The third case was *Re M*, a 24-year-old man who had been vegetative for 8 years since a severe head injury (44). He continued to suffer from epileptic seizures, one of which was witnessed during examination by the expert commissioned by the Official Solicitor. This expert also observed nystagmus in response to caloric stimulation. He regarded these two features as evidence of some cortical activity but not as evidence of consciousness. Both he and the expert for the Trust agreed that *M* was in PVS although breaching one of the 'other features' in the College guidelines. It is interesting in the light of the two previous cases that the letter from the Official Solicitor commissioning a report from his expert in this case had specifically stated that all the criteria of the College report did not have to be satisfied. The application was not opposed and the President granted the required declaration. This issue arose yet again in a recent case (45) when the judge stated that the International Working Party (p. 13) provided far more helpful guidelines than did the report of the Royal College.

What seems clear from these three cases is that the court was primarily concerned to hear experts testify that the patient had no awareness. If satisfied about this but there were some features that might indicate residual limited activity in the cerebral cortex it was prepared to grant a declaration to allow withdrawal of life-sustaining treatment. It was therefore unfortunate that the Law Commission in its recommendations chose to replace the term permanent vegetative state with the phrase 'has no activity in the cerebral cortex' (p. 156).

In October 2000, a few days after the Human Rights Act of 1998, reflecting the European Convention on Human Rights, became law in

England two vegetative cases were heard together by the President (now Dame Elizabeth Butler-Sloss). *Mrs H* had been vegetative since a cardiac arrest and, because she had a tube blockage, her case was brought urgently and was the first case to come to court in less than a year (8 months) after nontraumatic brain damage. *Mrs M* had been vegetative for more than 3 years since a cardiac arrest under anaesthesia. Neither case was controversial from a medical viewpoint. However, the major front page item in *The Guardian* newspaper a few days earlier (46) had predicted that the Official Solicitor might challenge the withdrawal of ANH as infringing Article 2 of the Act – that the right to life shall be protected by law. In the event, counsel for the two Trusts and counsel for the Official Solicitor each argued, using slightly different approaches, that the decisions in *Bland* and subsequent cases similar to that sought in these two cases did not infringe the Human Rights Act (47). The President agreed and granted the declarations.

Article 2 enjoins the State to refrain from taking life and to take appropriate steps to safeguard life. The latter positive obligation is less absolute than the negative one. States are left to decide what is appropriate to safeguard life and to resolve conflicts between this and other relevant rights (such as privacy and autonomy). This conflict was resolved in English Common Law for vegetative patients by the binding decision of the Lords in *Bland*, from which long extracts were quoted. An omission to treat was not culpable if there was no duty to act, and there was no such duty if such action was not in the best interests of the patient as objectively assessed. Not only was there no duty to treat, but there was no right to do so, if the treatment was not in the patient's best interests. There was no question of intentional killing within the meaning of the Act. The positive obligation to treat does not mandate futile treatment. The appropriateness of treatment might be defined as whatever was not negligent by the *Bolam* principle of being in accord with a responsible body of medical opinion.

Article 8 speaks to respect for the privacy and autonomy of the individual and for his family life. In the context of the vegetative patient, this Article could be regarded as mandating the withdrawal of treatment. One counsel considered that the principles applied in the Strasbourg court under Article 8 bore a resemblance to the approach of the House of Lords to the issue of medical consent in *Bland*. Article 3 prohibits inhuman or degrading treatment or punishment ('treatment' being used more broadly than medical). Indeed counsel for the Official Solicitor considered that it was unlikely that medical treatment given in good faith could ever be regarded as breaching this article. In any event, for the insensate vegetative patient he believed that neither providing nor withdrawing treatment could be regarded as inhuman or degrading. Counsel for the Trusts put the case for a more flexible approach to Article 3, allowing that persisting with futile treatment might involve its violation. Indeed, in granting a declaration for a vegetative patient in the English court earlier in 2000 a judge had regarded Article 3 as protecting the right to die in these circumstances (48).

Whilst noting that there had been no Strasbourg court decision on withdrawing ANH from a PVS patient, counsel for each side quoted liberally from court decisions in many other countries that echoed what was said in the *Bland* courts. These supported what one of the Law Lords in *Bland* had referred to as the growing international consensus on this issue. A private prosecution for passive euthanasia in Switzerland was the only case to have been brought under Article 2 concerning alleged failure to provide medical treatment that had resulted in death (49). The Commission had struck this out, maintaining that the law prohibiting negligent failure to treat was adequate to meet the State's positive obligation under Article 2. That case, together with the many court decisions allowing treatment withdrawal from vegetative patients but without specific reference to the Human Rights Act, could be regarded as giving persuasive support for the withdrawal of ANH from vegetative patients. Nothing in the case law of the Convention required the present court to depart from the House of Lords' analysis in *Bland*, according to counsel for the Trusts. He maintained that the distinction between acts and omissions in *Bland* was equally applicable to the distinction between positive and negative obligations under Article 2.

An attempt was made in this court by an antieuthanasia pressure group to present the case that withdrawal of ANH was against Articles 2 and 3 of the Act. This organization, ALERT (Against Legalized Euthanasia – Research and Teaching), was formed in 1991 when the *Bland* case was under discussion but not yet resolved. After reading a written witness statement and discussing the matter with counsel for each side in this case, the judge ruled that counsel for ALERT had no right of audience in her court as it was not a party to the case before her.

Review of the medical details of 16 PVS cases in the English court for which data are available shows that nine were aged 21–30 years, four from 36 to 49, and one of 81; one was a baby and in one the age was not known. Nontraumatic brain damage had occurred in 11. In four cases the feeding tube had blocked and in two ventilation was withdrawn. Duration of the vegetative state was 2 years or less in five, $2\frac{1}{2}$ to $4\frac{1}{2}$ (189) years in six cases and one each of 5, 8 and 9 years.

No PVS case has so far come to the English courts where it was claimed that there was a valid advance directive refusing ANH, but in *obiters* in more than one court it has been observed that the existence of one would be good reason to withdraw ANH. Indeed, it has been speculated that in such an event there would be no need to seek court approval for withdrawal. In practice, however, a court might be invited to judge the validity of the advance directive in the particular circumstances. Although there is no statute in Britain recognizing advance directives, it is held in common law that they have the same legal authority as a contemporaneous refusal by the patient. Not only would doctors be obliged to respect them but relatives and close associates of the patient would have no right to override them.

Delayed comment on the *Bland* decision

In spite of the lukewarm endorsement of the House of Lords Select Committee, and the lack of the legislative developments hoped for by the Law Lords, there has been no problem with the cases that have continued to go through the High Court, with the declaration sought being granted in every case. Moreover, the detailed arguments set out by counsel on both sides in response to the challenge of the Human Rights Act in October 2000 amount to an endorsement of the *Bland* decision and acknowledgement that similar decisions are being made in other jurisdictions. The European Commission research project in late 1994 sought medical opinions about the management of PVS patients. Of 1027 UK doctors who responded to a questionnaire, 79% believed that the *Bland* decision had been right and 11% that it was wrong (50). Only 14% agreed with the recommendation that future cases should all be required to go to court.

An editorial in the *British Medical Journal* in 1999 pointed out that Britain was the only country requiring court approval for the withdrawal of ANH from vegetative patients and questioned whether it might not be time to review this policy (51). It emphasized that several of the *Bland* judges had expressed the view that such a requirement should be for a trial period only and that the Law Commissions had both proposed alternative formalities that would avoid involving the courts. Only years later did the medical profession (the BMA Medical Ethics Committee) come up with proposed formalities for withdrawal of ANH that would apply not only to PVS cases but to other conditions as well and that were designed to avoid the need to go to court (p. 112). Indeed, in the updating of this guidance to take account of the Human Rights Act, concern was expressed that the requirement of judicial approval before withdrawing ANH from PVS patients, but not from other patients, could be regarded as discrimination that would violate Article 14 (52). This threat would be removed if it were no longer necessary to take PVS cases to court.

Immediate reactions from Catholic commentators to the *Bland* decision were confused but later reactions were adverse, concerned that it might seem to legitimize euthanasia and physician-assisted suicide (p. 117). An academic lawyer writing in a legal journal emphasized the ambiguities in the speeches of some of the judges (53). As the intention of withdrawing ANH was clearly to bring about the death of the patient, resulting in possible benefits to others – paying of life insurance, saving the costs of continued treatment and relieving the grief of visiting relatives – why was this not murder? It might be reasonable to limit treatment but not nourishment given by means needing no continuing medical skills. Denying the personhood of these invalids was breaking off human solidarity. There was a failure to distinguish between a person being subject to indignities and being in an undignified condition. Many people might be rescued from undignified conditions by benevolent but illegal termination of life. Without a clear defence of the principle of the sanctity of life, this principle had been sacrificed to that of self-determination. The tone of his final words contrasted with the measured judgements in the *Bland* courts – 'Civilised relationships should have no truck with choices intended to terminate the lives of innocent people'. However, the submission of the Catholic bishops to the House of Lords committee was very moderate, and indeed was made jointly with the bishops of the Church of England. It stated simply that there could be no blanket permission regarding complex issues such as withdrawing ANH from PVS patients but that every person's needs and rights must be dealt with on a case-to-case basis.

'Euthanasia by stages' was the title of an article in the legal pages of the *Lancet* some 4 years after *Bland* (54). It argued that euthanasia should not be looked on as a uniform whole because this led to blurred rhetoric and widespread distrust of the concept. Judges had not helped by declaring that treatment withdrawal was not euthanasia because no new external agent was involved, and by distinguishing between the right to die and the right to choose how to live, even when that choice made an early death likely. A legal vacuum was developing that demanded an urgent legislative response for certain situations, such as the vegetative state. If there was to be an end to the present trail of court decisions a medical code of practice was not good enough. These authors proposed a Medical Futility Bill to make it lawful to withdraw life-sustaining treatment if two suitably experienced doctors declared that the patient was in a permanent vegetative state. The article went on to suggest a modification of the Suicide Act of 1961 to allow physician-assisted suicide for competent patients with progressive paralysing neurological disorders who were unable to end their own lives without assistance.

Following the first vegetative case in the Scottish Court of Session (p. 168), another Scottish academic lawyer (McLean) made a further plea for legislation (55). She pointed out that there was a massive paradox in the law. It would not allow doctors to assist the deaths of competent patients who had decided that it was not in their best interest to go on living, but it could authorize doctors to withdraw life-sustaining treatment from patients whose wishes could not be known. The latter was justified on the basis of best interests, but vegetative patients by definition had no interests, so how could it be decided what was best for them? Decisions about best interests were therefore at best speculative and at worst actually the interests of others. She went on: 'In our fear of addressing the possibility that there might be conditions which made death preferable to life, and to avoid confronting the euthanasia debate, we had developed tests (of best interests) that were philosophically and ethically flawed in order that the "right" decision could be made'. Nor, once the decision had been made that death was the best option for a vegetative patient, did we allow the most dignified way of bringing this about. Rather than leaving these matters to a series of one-off *ad hoc* judgements, there was need for a legislative framework. This should concede that sanctity of life was not absolute, and provide guidelines that led to consistent, accountable, transparent decisions.

This same commentator returned to this issue 3 years later in a medical journal (56). She maintained that because of the ethical and legal commitment to the sanctity of life the law had been led to disingenuous and unhelpful approaches to the problem of vegetative patients. The law was effectively endorsing nonvoluntary euthanasia but dressing it up as something else. She went on: 'We should overcome our reluctance to admit that the intention of these decisions was to bring about the patient's death, and then to find an ethically and legally satisfactory route to permitting this to happen'. 'We needed', she maintained, 'to review all end-of-life decisions so that doctors could exercise their judgement without fear of legal reprisal, and that patients and their families could be treated with compassion'. The alternative, that would benefit no one, would be to decide that such decisions should never be taken.

The Scottish case

Scottish law has always been distinctly different from English law and with different names for its courts and law officers. The practice notes of the Official Solicitor do not apply to Scotland but rulings from the House of Lords do. As a result, the previous relaxed attitude to withdrawal of ANH in 1991 (p. 148) could no longer apply when another case arose in 1995. It resulted in an application for a declaration from the Court of Session (Scotland's highest civil court) at the end of 1995. Mrs. Johnstone aged 52 had been vegetative for 4 years following nontraumatic brain damage and the application to withdraw ANH was supported by all the members of her family (57). It was opposed by the court appointed *curator ad litem* and by the Lord Advocate, Scotland's Chief Criminal Law Officer. As this case would be the first of its kind to be dealt with under Scottish law and the judgement would decide how future cases would be dealt with, the judge of first instance (the Lord Ordinary) in the Outer House felt that he needed guidance. He therefore referred it to the Inner House of the Court of Session, where the Lord President (Scotland's senior Civil Judge) appointed four other judges to consider the matter with him. In effect, this was rather as though in *Bland* the House of Lords had been asked for guidance before the first judgement rather than its going there on appeal.

The Lord President opened the unanimous judgement of the Inner House by observing that doctors might decide about clinical features but they could not assume the lawfulness of treatment withdrawal on the grounds that it accorded with accepted medical ethics. As recommended by the Scottish Law Commission, doctors were entitled to look to the courts to reassure them, in the absence of a declaration by Parliament. He observed that the Scottish court retained the power of *parens patriae* that the *Bland* judges regretted that they did not have. It would therefore be appropriate to use this in such cases to authorize a given line of action. This would have the same authority as consent given by the patient. However, in this case, where evidence had already been led, it was unreasonable to require the parties to begin a new application with the attendant delay and expense, and therefore a declaration could be made. However, in response to the Lord Advocate's assertion that a civil court could not declare in advance that a given action would not be criminal, the declaration should make clear that it applied only to civil law – in the hope that in practice no prosecution would follow. It would therefore offer less protection to doctors than the *Bland* rulings did, until some other solution was found to reassure them.

As for the merits of the case, these judges found the arguments in *Bland* persuasive and they quoted extensively from the speeches in the House of Lords. They also noted that other common law jurisdictions had found similarly. They found that there was no benefit in prolonging the life of Mrs. Johnstone, as this was of no benefit to her, and was therefore not in her best interests. Future cases could be dealt with by a petition to the Court of Session to authorize treatment withdrawal. There should be two medical reports confirming that the case was compliant with the BMA guidelines. The court would appoint a *curator ad litem* with powers to commission a further medical report. The cases would normally be heard in chambers but there was no recommendation about maintaining the privacy of the parties. The judgement went on: 'nothing in this opinion is intended to suggest that an application must be made in every case'. Shortly after this judgement was handed down, the Lord Advocate issued a policy statement to the effect that he would guarantee immunity to every doctor who discontinued ANH on the authorization of the Court of Session. A legal commentator later wrote that, in spite of the ruling that not every case need come to court, the prudent doctor would likely seek such court approval, thus making practice effectively the same as in England (55). However, this ruling gave more specific protection to doctors than applied in England. The Inner House concluded that the Outer House was competent to decide such cases, and it authorized the Lord Ordinary to deal with this case in the light of the guidance it had provided. He granted the declarator a month later.

The Adults with Incapacity (Scotland) Act 2000 provides for the court to appoint a proxy decision maker for an incapacitated patient over the age of

16. There was a legal obligation to 'take account of' the views of such a proxy, but it was for the doctor to make the final decision. If there was disagreement between the treating doctor and the proxy, then the Mental Welfare Commission should be asked to nominate another doctor to give a second opinion. If this agreed with the treating doctor, the treatment could be provided regardless of the view of the proxy. A court could always be asked for a determination if there was serious disagreement. This Act is primarily about decisions to provide treatment, not withholding or withdrawing, but the court's inherent jurisdiction could cover such limitation of treatment.

REFERENCES

1 Bayliss RIS. Thou shalt not strive officiously. *BMJ* 1982; 285: 1373–5

2 Rouse F. The *Cruzan* case. *Lancet* 1991; 337: 105–6

3 Institute of Medical Ethics Working Party. Withdrawal of life-support from patients in a persistent vegetative state. *Lancet* 1991; 337: 96–8

4 Jennett B, Dyer C. Persistent vegetative state and the right to die: the United States and Britain. *BMJ* 1991; 302: 1256–8

5 Gillon R. Living wills, powers of attorney and medical practice. *J Med Ethics* 1988; 14: 59–60

6 *In re F (Mental patient; sterilisation)* [1990] 2 A.C. 1

7 Hamilton D. Dilemma of the twilight victims. *Sunday Express* 1991: 1 Dec

8 Medical Ethics Committee of the British Medical Association. *Discussion paper on patients in a persistent vegetative state.* London: BMA, 1992

9 *Bolam* v. *Friern Hospital Management Committee* [1957] 1 W.L.R. 582

10 In *re C (A minor. Wardship: medical treatment) [1990] Fam. 26*

11 In *re J (A minor. Wardship: medical treatment) [1991] Fam. 33*

12 *Airedale NHS Trust* v. *Bland* [1993] 1 All ER 821

13 Jennett B. Letting vegetative patients die: ethical and lawful and brings Britain into line. *BMJ* 1992; 305: 1305–6

14 Andrews K. Letting vegetative patients die (letter). *BMJ* 1992; 305: 1506

15 Fergusson A. Letting vegetative patients die (letter). *BMJ* 1992; 305: 1506

16 Cole AP. Letting vegetative patients die. *BMJ* 1992; 306 (letter): 142–3

17 Budd C. *Euthanasia and hard cases.* London: CatholicMedia Office, 1992

18 McQueen M, Walsh JL. Comment on the Bland case. *The Tablet* 1992; 19/26 December

19 Kelly K. Comment on the Bland case. *The Tablet* 1993; 13 March

20 Puxon M. Mercy without certainty. *Lancet* 1992; 340: 1343

21 Brahams D. Persistent vegetative state. *Lancet* 1992; 340: 1534–5

22 Anon. A 'life' no longer supported. *Lancet* 1993; 341: 410

23 House of Lords. *Report of Select Committee on Medical Ethics.* HL 21–1. London: HMSO, 1994

24 Royal College of Physicians. Report on the permanent vegetative state. *J R Coll Physicians Lond* 1996; 30: 119–21

25 BMA Medical Ethics Committee. *Withholding and withdrawing life-prolonging medical treatment.* London: BMJ Books, 1999.

26 Law Commission. *Mentally incapacitated adults and decision-making; medical treatment and research.* Consultation paper 129. London, Law Commission, 1993.

27 Official Solicitor to the Supreme Court. *Practice note: vegetative state.* [1994] All ER 242

28 Official Solicitor to the Supreme Court. *Practice note: vegetative state.* [1996] 2 FLR 375

29 Law Commission. *Mental incapacity. Report 231.* London; Law Commission, 1995

30 Scottish Law Commission. *Report on incapable adults.* (No. 151) Edinburgh; Scottish Law Commission, 1995

31 Lord Chancellor's Department. *Making decisions. Command 4465,* London, HMSO, 1999.

32 Hinchliffe M. Vegetative state patients. *NLJ Practitioner* 1996; 1 November: 1579–80, 85

33 *Frenchay Healthcare NHS Trust* v. *S* [1994] 1 WLR 601

34 Stone J. Withholding life-sustaining treatment: the ultimate decision. *New Law J* 1994; 144: 205–6

35 *Swindon and Marlborough NHS Trust* v. *S* [1995] Med Law Rev 84

36 *Re G (Adult Patient: Publicity)* [1995] 2 FLR 528

37 *Re C (Adult Patient: Restriction of publicity after death)* [1996] 1 FCR 605

38 *Re G (Persistent Vegetative State)* [1995] 2 FCR 46

39 *Re C (A baby)* [1996] 2 FLR 43

40 *Re D* [1998] 1 FLR 411

41 Dyer C. PVS criteria put under spotlight. *BMJ* 1997; 314: 919

42 Brahams D. UK judge allows withdrawal of artificial feeding in prolonged non-PVS coma. *Lancet* 1997; 349: 932

43 *Re H (adult: incompetent)* [1998] 38 BMLR 11

44 *Re M* [1998] Unreported extract from LEXUS

45 *NHS Trust* v. *H* [2001] All ER (D) 363

46 Dyer C. Court test for new right to life law. *The Guardian* 2000, 1 Oct

47 *NHS Trust A* v. *hus M and NHS Trust B* v. *hus H* [2001] All ER 801

48 *NHS* v. *D* (Unreported) Cazalet J, 5 July 2000

49 *Widmer* v. *Switzerland* (Application No. 20527/92, Unreported)

50 Grubb A, Walsh P, Lambe N et al. Survey of British clinicians' views on

management of patients in persistent vegetative state. *Lancet* 1996; 348: 35–40

51 Jennett B. Should cases of permanent vegetative state still go to court? *BMJ* 1999; 319: 786–7

52 BMA Medical Ethics Committee. *Withholding and withdrawing life-prolonging medical treatment* 2nd ed. London: BMJ Books, 2001

53 Finnis JM. *Bland:* crossing the Rubicon? *Law Q Rev* 1993; 109: 329–37

54 Mason JK, Mulligan D. Euthanasia by stages. *Lancet* 1996; 347: 810–11

55 McLean S. End-of-life decisions and the law. *J Med Ethics* 1996; 22: 261–2

56 McLean S. Legal and ethical aspects of the vegetative state. *J Clin Pathol* 1999; 52: 490–93

57 *Law Hospital NHS Trust* v. *Lord Advocate and others.* 39 BMLR 166 (1998)

11

Legal issues in other countries

South Africa

The case of *Clarke* was decided in July 1992 (1) and was referred to a few months later by more than one judge in the *Bland* courts in England. This 68-year-old doctor had been in a vegetative state for 4 years since a cardiac arrest and had a living will (details p. 204). His wife and family applied to the court to appoint her as *curatrix personae* with powers to discontinue nasogastric feeding. The court-appointed *curator ad litem* did not oppose the application but the Attorney General for the Province did. The judge ruled that there was no reason why a curator should not have power to give effect to the valid prior direction of the patient to be allowed to die. He quoted *Quinlan* and *Re J* and *Re B* in support of his decision to grant the application.

New Zealand

The case of *L* was decided in August 1992 (2) and, although not a classical vegetative state due to brain damage, it was extensively quoted by the *Bland* judges later that year, and by judges in other jurisdictions since. He was a 59-year-old man with severe Guillain–Barre syndrome which affected the peripheral nerves and gradually paralysed all the muscles in his body (details p. 206). For the last year he had been dependent on a ventilator and unable to interact in any way with his surroundings and displayed no awareness. The treating doctor, supported by the patient's wife, sought a declaration from the court that it would not be unlawful to withdraw ventilation. The Attorney General opposed this. In granting the declaration the judge referred to the case of *Nancy B* who also had severe Guillain–Barre but was competent to request removal of her respirator, which the

Quebec Superior Court had allowed (3). He also referred to *Re J*, the badly handicapped infant in the English court where it was said that a doctor was not under a duty to prolong life if this was not, in his judgement, in the best interests of the patient. The issue of treatment withdrawal in these circumstances was essentially a medical one which could not be resolved by strict logic, and certainly not by legal logic. In making a declaratory order, in this case the judge hoped that this would encourage doctors to reach such decisions in future without recourse to the courts.

In 1993, the Medical Council of New Zealand received a report on withdrawal of ANH from vegetative patients that it had commissioned from a University Bioethics Research Centre (4). This recommended that withdrawal of ANH was appropriate once permanence was declared and considered that this could be done in a matter of months, but in less than a year. The decision to withdraw should be taken jointly by the medical team and the family, with advice from a local ethical committee if there were difficulties. Recourse to a court of law was regarded as undesirable. It recommended, however, that the Law Commission should prepare a report and draft legislation to recognize the validity of living wills and enduring powers of attorney. For patients without such prior arrangements, the law should permit a decision to withdraw treatment to be made by a proxy on the basis of substituted judgment whenever possible. Failing this, the doctor should decide on the basis of best interests as judged in conjunction with an Ethics Committee. The following year, the New Zealand Medical Association issued a policy statement (5) effectively endorsing this report and the Medical Council saw no need to add a statement of its own. It seems that no legislation has been developed and no cases have gone to court. A book on *Health Care and the Law* in 2000 noted that the right to refuse treatment was enshrined in the New Zealand Bill of Rights Act and in the Code of Health and Disability Service Consumers Rights (6). It also asserted that it was accepted that no one was required to prolong life by extraordinary means. Based on this principle, medical decisions that could be interpreted as leading to passive euthanasia were frequently made, and although these were potential offences no prosecutions were laid. This book quoted from *Bland, Re B* and the *Auckland* case but made no mention of incompetent patients in general or the vegetative state in particular. In 2000 the Medical Council included in the update of its handbook for doctors *Good Medical Practice* (7) a note that a request for withdrawal of ANH from a permanently vegetative patient, either from the family or via an advance directive, should be respected.

Republic of Ireland

The Republic of Ireland, like the USA and several other European countries, has a written constitution defining a number of rights to which its citizens are entitled. These resemble those enshrined in the European Convention of Human Rights that became law in England in October 2000. In the *Ward of Court* PVS case in the Irish High Court in 1995 (8) many of the arguments used were similar to those subsequently used in the English High Court in October 2000. It was successfully argued there that withdrawal of ANH from vegetative patients did not infringe the Human Rights Act (p. 162). Another feature of Ireland is that over 90% of the population are Roman Catholic and the Church has always had considerable influence over affairs of State in Ireland. It is one of the few European countries where abortion remains illegal, and there is particular sensitivity about euthanasia. In this case, moral theologians appeared on both sides with conflicting arguments about the moral acceptability of withdrawing ANH.

The *Ward of Court* was a woman of 45 years who had been vegetative for 23 years since an anaesthetic accident (details p. 214). Her family was frustrated by the unwillingness of the doctors and nuns responsible for her care to limit life-sustaining treatment or the use of antibiotics. When an anaesthetic was given to replace her gastrostomy tube for the second time, an application was made to court to order withdrawal of ANH. This was opposed by the hospice treating her, by her *guardian ad litem* and by the Attorney General. Their arguments were that withdrawal would infringe her right to life under the Irish Constitution, that she was not terminally ill and that ANH was not medical treatment. She had some tracking eye movements which led opponents of the application to claim that she was completely different from *Bland*. The judge ruled that she was near vegetative, and that as she had been a Ward of Court for many years the court could use its *parens patriae* powers to decide about her treatment. He ruled that ANH was medical treatment that could lawfully be withdrawn, and that this would be in her best interests. An appeal to the Supreme Court was dismissed in a four to one decision.

The Irish Council for Civil Liberties welcomed the decision but

Table 11.1. Physicians' attitudes to court decision approving withdrawal of ANH – was it/would it be right?

	Court case	n	Yes[a]	No[a]	DK[a]
United Kingdom	*Bland*	1027	79	11	7
Netherlands	*Stinissen*	275	78	6	13
Ireland	*Ward of Court*	15	47	53	0
Ireland	If fully PVS	15	60	33	7
Belgium	If PVS 3 yrs	208	52	30	16
Germany	If PVS 3 yrs	283	33	43	18
France	If PVS 3 yrs	50	14	66	14
Greece	If PVS 3 yrs	153	45	31	22

[a]Percentage of physicians answering yes, no or don't know (DK) about a previous court case in their country; if no such case, if their national court were to approve withdrawal after 3 years in PVS. For Ireland, where the Ward was deemed to have been nearly vegetative, they were asked also for their opinion if the Ward had been fully vegetative.
From European Biomedical survey (9).

statements from the Irish Medical Council and the Nursing Board of Ireland asserted that ANH was a basic human need and implied that the participation of professionals in carrying out the court's order might lead to disciplinary action. This was a reversal of the more usual situation when doctors and nurses who wish to withdraw treatment are unwilling to do so for fear of legal repercussions. Here, the corporate professional bodies were unwilling to let doctors and nurses proceed even though they had been given the protection and the authority of the law. Eventually, a doctor and some nurses volunteered to help and she died at home almost two months after the Supreme Court decision. No action was taken against the professionals involved.

The European study of physicians' attitudes (9,10) included only 15 responding Irish doctors (of 25 invited). Only 47% of them agreed or strongly agreed with the decision about the Ward of Court, but this rose to 60% if they had been assured that she was fully vegetative (Table 11.1). Asked about future policy, only 14% felt that each case should go to court; the preferred option was for the doctor and family to decide, with many fewer than in most other countries favouring either legislation or guidelines (Table 11.2).

Table 11.2. Doctors' views on future policy on making decision to withdraw ANH

	n	Option			
		1	2	3	4
United Kingdom	1027	14	39	54	78
Netherlands	275	4	34	44	68
Ireland	15	14	54	33	27
Belgium	208	10	49	40	57
Germany	283	12	20	28	57
France	50	10	20	22	24
Greece	153	10	33	36	61

Figures show percentage agreeing or strongly agreeing when asked about each option in turn: Option 1, every case to court; Option 2, doctor decides with family; Option 3, enact a law to allow doctor to decide with family; Option 4, enact a law to allow doctor to decide with family in accordance with guidelines.
From European Biomedical survey (9).

As well as having a written constitution, Ireland has, like several other European countries, a code of ethical conduct, in this case published by the Medical Council of Ireland (11). It was this document that the Medical Council relied on when issuing its statement after the conclusion of the *Ward of Court* case. Its 1994 edition included a translation from the French of the Principles of Medical Ethics in Europe adopted by the Conference Internationale des Ordres et des Organismes d'Attributions Similaires, Paris on 6 January 1987, which the Council fully supported. Its Article 12 on the Care of the Terminally Ill recommended only that interventions be restricted to such treatments as were appropriate to preserve the quality of life and to permit the patient to retain his dignity, but neither ANH nor the vegetative state were mentioned. There has been no updating of the medical or nursing codes since then and no other cases have come to court.

Netherlands

The case of *Mrs Stinissen* provoked wide publicity about the issue of withdrawal of ANH from a permanently vegetative patient. In 1974, when aged 32, she suffered an anaesthetic accident during Caesarean section leaving her in a vegetative state. After 11 years her husband considered her condition to be hopeless and wished her to die, but the doctors in the nursing home were unwilling to discuss the matter with him, and refused to let him take her home. They held vitalist views based on religious conviction. This was, therefore, rather similar to the case in Ireland (p. 175). Her husband briefed journalists in order to bring the matter to public attention and a book was published about the case. Two years later (1987), the case came to court but the application was unsuccessful (12). Three years later (1990), after the intervention of the Professor of Ethics at the Protestant Free University of Amsterdam, legal consent to withdraw treatment was given. The Dutch Association for Patients (a pro-life organization) brought a civil action to force the doctors to continue feeding. The District Court ruled that it had no standing in the case and this was supported by the Court of Appeal. She eventually died following withdrawal of treatment, after 17 years in a vegetative state.

In 1991, the Dutch Medical Association published an interim report on the management of vegetative patients (13) and the Ministry of Health then set up a wide ranging committee under the Health Council of the Netherlands. This comprised doctors from many specialities, ethicists and lawyers and it reported in 1994 (14). It stated that the mere existence of a body was not a human life and that these patients when healthy would have considered that living in this state was extremely undesirable. It was morally justifiable to withdraw life-prolonging treatment. ANH was regarded as one such medical treatment that could be withdrawn once the vegetative state had been declared permanent (12 months after trauma, 6 months for other cases).

This report stated that the family should play an important but never the decisive role in making the decision to withdraw treatment. Netherlands is the only European country to legislate for a patient to nominate a proxy for health decision making, but doctors may override a surrogate's decision that is considered not in the patient's best interests (10). An advance directive would be important in making a decision, and again Netherlands is the only European country that legally requires a doctor to comply with a valid, written directive. There was no mention in the Health Council report about active termination of life, as this would go against the euthanasia regulations that require the patient to actively request this over a period of time. Nor was there any mention of involving the courts in decisions to withdraw ANH and no further court cases seem to have been reported. The

European study of physician's attitudes found 78% of Dutch doctors approving the final decision of the *Stinissen* case (Table 11.1). In regard to future policy only 4% were in favour of having the courts decide, while 68% wished to see legislation allowing doctors and families to decide in accordance with agreed guidelines (Table 11.2).

Germany

The case of *Schwatza* was a woman of 71 years who had had irreversible brain damage for 3 years following cardiac arrest. The family doctor proposed that ANH be withdrawn and the son reluctantly agreed. There was no written advance directive but her son remembered that during the viewing of a TV programme on intensive care she had said she did not want to end up like that. The staff refused to withdraw treatment and reported the matter to the guardianship court, who reported it to the prosecutors. She lived for many months before dying of complications. After her death, a regional criminal court in Bavaria convicted the doctor and the patient's son of attempted manslaughter, arguing that the law required a written directive before withdrawing ANH; both were fined. However, the Federal High Court in 1994 ruled that a guardian could take such a decision if there was sufficient evidence for the presumed will of the patient and it referred the case back to the first court (15,16). At the retrial, several witnesses testified to the patient having made statements on many occasions about not wishing such treatment to be continued in a situation such as this, and the court set aside its original conviction and punishment. This case was said to have marginally extended the interpretation of German laws on the borderline between criminal homicide and legal passive euthanasia, and it provoked contrasting reactions from medical commentators. It led to the widespread acceptance of living wills in Germany and to statements supporting the resolution of this case, according to a recent review (17). This quotes an interview with the President of the Supreme Court in 1997 when he declared that the prohibition of killing on request (euthanasia) should not impede respecting a patient's will not to be subjected to life-prolonging measures. In 1998, the German Medical Association guidelines stated that, in the absence of an expressed will from the patient or guardian, a doctor must act in accordance with the presumed will of the patient (however reconstructed).

The Frankfurt case concerned an 85-year-old woman who had been in a 'persistent coma' for some months since a stroke and was not expected to improve. A local court appointed her daughter as her care assistant, who then applied to the Guardianship Court to withdraw ANH in accordance with the wishes of her mother, who had not wanted a protracted death (18). The original lower court refused this, claiming that the relevant section of the Civil Code did not apply when the aim was to bring about death. On appeal, this decision was upheld by the District Court. However, the Higher Regional Court of Appeal in July 1998 (7 months after the stroke) considered that withdrawal of ANH was permissible if it was the presumed will of the patient and had been approved by the Guardianship Court. Although it stated that the ethical guidelines from the Federal Medical Council on the care of the dying could not be applied directly to vegetative patients, because they were not dying, the presumed will of the vegetative patient might allow treatment withdrawal. It ruled that the articles of the German Constitution (or Basic Law) that referred to the right to dignity, liberty and self-determination took priority over the right to life. Withdrawal of treatment was not a form of passive euthanasia but rather an aid to dying. A high standard of evidence of the patient's presumed will was required as it was the patient's interests that mattered, not someone else's opinion of these. It did not specify what form that evidence might take, but a care assistant was held qualified to give evidence of the patient's will. The care assistant had the legal authority to further the patient's interests, including decisions about prolonging life. The sensitivity of these issues in Germany is highlighted by the national outcry against the decision in the Frankfurt case, and this resulted in the patient's daughter deciding not to go ahead with the treatment withdrawal, despite the court having approved this.

In a lengthy commentary on the Frankfurt case, with references to previous American, English, Irish and Scottish cases, a German academic lawyer drew attention to the influence of Germany's troubled past on current practice (19). The concept of care assistants arose as an attempt to ensure that the patient had a voice, and that too much was not left to judges and doctors – both of whom had been complicit in the 1930s with the Nazi euthanasia programme for those 'unworthy of life'. Care assistants were, however, initially used mostly in decisions about the sterilization of mentally handicapped women and would appear to be the equivalent of a guardian in other jurisdictions.

In regard to vegetative patients, the European survey found many fewer doctors in Germany willing to consider withdrawing ANH than in other countries (p. 119). Only 33% would consider a legal decision to authorize this as right, 43% that it would be wrong (Table 11.1). Only 12% were in favour of such decisions being made by a court, and 57% would prefer legislation that allowed doctors and families to decide in accordance with guidelines (Table 11.2).

Other European countries

There is no case law in other countries of Europe. However, as a review of the legal scene in Europe points out (10), most of them have a written constitution, the articles of which specify various rights, most of which are reiterated in the European Convention of Human Rights. The application of these to the problem of withdrawing treatment from vegetative patients has been the subject of legal argument in the courts in England (p. 162), Ireland (p. 175) and Germany (p. 180). These would likely inform decision making in other countries where there is no relevant case law. Several countries also have codes of ethical conduct drawn up by medical associations or licensing councils, and several of these have guidelines for the care of the dying. These are mostly written in general terms of not persisting with futile treatment but do not specify either vegetative patients or withdrawal of ANH. A doctor failing to comply with these codes might risk disciplinary procedures being taken against him by the relevant authority. Only in France and Greece do these ethical codes for doctors have the force of law.

A recent report on withholding and withdrawing life support in intensive care units in **France** noted that this was prohibited by French legislation and that there were no guidelines from scientific bodies (20). None the less, this study revealed that decisions to limit life support were frequently taken by doctors in over 100 intensive care units in France. It may be significant that this paper was published in a British medical journal. There is less regard for patient autonomy in France where medical paternalism persists and the courts have never become involved in medical decisions (p. 119). Although doctors are supposed to respect the will of the patient, including refusal of treatment, they frequently see this as incompatible with their obligation to save life. There is almost no discussion in the legal literature about advance refusals or refusal by a proxy and the courts are very reluctant to become involved in medical decisions (17).

French physicians were reluctant to participate in the European study on vegetative patients. Of the 50 who eventually did make returns many fewer would ever consider withdrawing ANH than in other countries – 14% vs. the European average of 57%; this was fewer even than in Germany (8). Many fewer French doctors would consider a legal decision in favour of this as right (Table 11.1), and many fewer favoured legislation to allow doctors and families to decide about treatment withdrawal (Table 11.2).

In **Belgium** the criminal code specifies that it is a duty not to intentionally withhold food or care from people unable to look after themselves, and not to negligently withhold such care. However, the Belgian code of medical ethics states that only comfort care need be provided for a patient in deep unconsciousness – which could be taken to include vegetative patients. Moreover, Belgium is one of the few countries outside the USA that has produced a specific ethical code approving the withdrawal of ANH from vegetative patients (p. 118). Other countries that have produced such codes are the UK, the Netherlands and New Zealand. In spite of this, only 52% of Belgian doctors thought a court decision to allow withdrawal of ANH would be right (Table 11.1), and 57% supported legislation to allow doctors and families to decide in accordance with guidelines – the same number as in Germany (Table 11.2).

The conservative ethical attitude to this problem in **Mediterranean countries** has been described (p. 120) and there appears to have been no formal legal discussion of these issues in those countries. In **Scandinavia**, by contrast, there seems to be acceptance that treatment withdrawal from vegetative patients is covered by general statements from medical authorities about not persisting with futile treatment in dying patients (p. 118). In Denmark the right to refuse treatment is explicitly recognized by statute law, which states that a physician may refrain from beginning or continuing measures whose only effect is to postpone death. There is also a law on living wills and there is a Living Will Register that doctors can consult when deciding about a particular patient (17).

Canada

The Law Commission in 1983 recommended that a physician should not incur any criminal liability if he decides to discontinue or not to initiate treatment for an incompetent person when that treatment is no longer therapeutically useful and is not in the patient's best interests (21). This was referred to with approval by two of the judges in the *Bland* appeals courts. They also referred to the Quebec case of *Nancy B*, paralysed with Guillain–Barre disease, whose petition to be allowed to have a respirator withdrawn was granted – but she was competent, making it of limited relevance to a PVS case. A Canadian commentator in 1994 noted that in matters of law Canada sits uneasily on a fence between the English and American systems (22). Codes of ethics, such as that of the Canadian Medical Association, are silent on specifics, as was the Law Commission mentioned above. There are no Federal or Provincial ethics bodies (except for human research) but some hospitals have ethics committees and codes which seem to assume that ANH can be withdrawn. The assumption of this author was that such decisions are probably made by doctors after consultation with families and perhaps with advice from a hospital ethics committees. That no cases had come to court might indicate that the present situation was satisfactory, although doctors were acting in a legal limbo with the assumption that what seems to be moral is probably not illegal. However, the protection of doctors from legal liability was thereby discretionary rather than statutory.

Australia

There is no specific legislation dealing with vegetative patients and there appear to have been no court cases. However, between 1988 and 1993, a number of States passed Acts to respect the prior wishes of incompetent patients to refuse treatment, or to allow proxies to decide on refusal in order to protect them from futile treatment. In 1993 a lawyer reviewed the Australian position in the light of the *Bland*, New Zealand and American cases (23). He believed that the Australian legal lacuna was likely to be filled to a significant degree by the *Bland* case, from which he quoted extensively. Noting the reference in that case to the protection of the sanctity of human life by Article 2 of the European Convention, he observed that this corresponded to Article 6 of the International Convention of Civil and Political Rights, to which both Australia and New Zealand were signatories. He saw some difficulty for Australian courts in relying (as the *Bland* courts had) on generally accepted medical opinion as a guide to appropriate action, because in 1992 the High Court in Australia had rejected the use of the *Bolam* test (24).

He noted that the guidelines on *Dying with Dignity*, published by the New South Wales Health Department in 1993 (25), would likely affect the Australian approach to this issue. These allowed for a patient-advocate (effectively a patient-nominated surrogate) to be involved when the question of withholding or withdrawing futile treatment arose in a patient unable to refuse treatment by reason of incompetence and who had no advance directive. Moreover, it categorized maintaining the life of a permanently vegetative patient as futile. It recommended a decision based on best interests, in deciding which due account should be taken of any evidence of the patient's views and values – in effect allowing an element of substituted judgement to play a part. He concluded that existing legislation in Australia embraces the delegalizing orientation articulated in the *Quinlan* decision. After consultation with the family, responsibility remains with the treating doctor who has wide discretion to act in the best interests of the vegetative patient. He noted that Australia had not so far adopted the English practice of resolving doctors' difficulties in deciding about treatment withdrawal by declaratory orders in court, but an application to court might well be prudent for a doctor facing unusual circumstances in such a case.

An Australian textbook on law and medical practice in 1998 included a section on withdrawal of futile treatment (26). This again quoted extensively from the *Bland* case, and also mentioned the New Zealand and some American cases. With no similar case yet in the Australian courts there was no judicial authority on this issue, but it was likely that a court would take a view similar to that of judges in these other jurisdictions. Best interests of the patient was the key to such a decision, and determining them was the responsibility of the patient's doctors acting in accordance with good medical practice.

The New South Wales Supreme Court heard a case in December 2000 (27), when a relative challenged a medical decision to withdraw treatment from a 37-year-old man only a week after a cardiac arrest. In the following 3 weeks two neurologists declared him to be in chronic vegetative state. By

2 months he was fully conscious and moving all limbs. Referring to the situation in Britain, the judge observed that there was clear need in Australia for clear criteria for the diagnosis of the permanent vegetative state and the circumstances in which treatment might be withdrawn. The result was that the Commonwealth Health Minister requested the National Health and Medical Research Council to set up a committee to respond to this demand.

REFERENCES

1 *Clarke* v. *Hurst* Supreme Court of South Africa (Durban and Coast Local Division) July 1992

2 *Auckland Health Board* v. *Attorney-General (Re L)* [1993] 1 NZLR 2353

3 *Nancy B* v. *Hotel-Dieu de Quebec* [1992] 86 DLR (4th) 385

4 Bioethics Research Centre, University of Otago. *Persistent vegetative state and the withdrawal of food and fluids.* Report for the Medical Council of New Zealand, February 1993

5 New Zealand Medical Association. *Policy paper: persistent vegetative state.* Wellington: New Zealand Medical Association, 1994

6 Johnson S Ed. *Health Care and the Law* 2nd edn. Wellington, Brookers, 2000

7 Medical Council of New Zealand. *Good medical practice.* Wellington: Medical Council of New Zealand. 2000

8 *A Ward of Court* [1995] 2 IRLM 401

9 Grubb A, Walsh P, Lambe N et al. *The moral and legal issues surrounding the treatment and care of patients in the persistent vegetative state.* Report to European Biomedical and Health Research Programme, 1997 [on file in the library of the Centre of Medical Law and Ethics, King's College, London]

10 Grubb A, Walsh P, Lambe N. Reporting on the persistent vegetative state in Europe. *Med Law Rev* 1998; 6: 161–210

11 The Medical Council of Ireland. *A guide to ethical conduct and behaviour and to fitness to practise*, 4th edn. Dublin: Medical Council of Ireland, 1994

12 *Stinissen case* Jurisprudentie nr 1990/18. *Tijdschr Gezondheidsr* 1990; 14: 286–8

13 Dutch Medical Association. *Discussienota Levensbeeindigend handelen bij wilsonbekwame patienten. Deel 2: Langdurig comateuze patienten.* KNMG, Utrecht, Netherlands, 1991

14 Health Council of the Netherlands. *Patients in a vegetative state.* The Hague: Health Council of the Netherlands, 1994

15 Schwatza BGH 13 Sep 94 1 Str 357/94, BGHST 40, 257

16 Koch H-G, Bernat E, Meisel A. Self-determination, privacy and the right to die: a

comparative analysis. *Eur J Health Law* 1997; 4: 127–43

17 Nys H. Physician involvement in a patient's death: a continental European perspective. *Med Law Rev* 1999; 7: 208–46

18 OLG Frankfurt, a.M. 20 W. 224/98, N.J.W. 1998, 2749

19 Aziz M. The role of care assistants in the withdrawal of hydration and nutrition in Germany. *Med Leg Rev* 1999; 7: 307–26

20 Ferrand E, Robert R, Ingrand P et al. Withholding and withdrawal of life support in intensive-care units in France: a prospective survey. *Lancet* 2001; 357: 9–14

21 Canadian Law Commission. *Report on euthanasia, aiding suicide and cessation of treatment. Report 20.* Ottawa, 1983

22 Emson HE. The right to die: withdrawal of tube feeding in the persistent vegetative state in Canada. In *Decision-making and problems of incompetence.* Grubb A (Ed). Chichester: John Wiley & Sons, 1994. 181–6

23 Freckelton I. Withdrawal of life support: the 'persistent vegetative state' conundrum. *J Law Med* 1993; 1: 35–46

24 *Rogers* v. *Whitaker* [1992] 175 CLR 479; 109 ALR 625

25 New South Wales Health Department. *Dying with dignity: interim guidelines on management.* Sydney, 1993

26 Skene L. *Law and medical practice; rights, duties, claims and defences.* London: Butterworths, 1998

27 *Northridge* v. *Central Sydney Area Health Service* [2000] NSWSC 1241

12

Details of some landmark legal cases

The main legal issues arising from each of these cases have already been dealt with in previous chapters but the accounts here include fuller details. References to significant commentaries on each case are given. The cases are in the chronological order of the final judgements as in many instances these included references to previous judgements, often in other jurisdictions. The cases given in detail here are as follows:

Karen Quinlan New Jersey 1976	p. 187
Clarence Herbert (*Barber*) California 1983	190
Claire Conroy New Jersey 1985	192
Paul Brophy Massachusetts 1986	194
Mary O'Connor New York 1988	196
Nancy Cruzan Missouri 1988, US Supreme 1990	198
Frederick Cyril Clarke South Africa 1992	204
'*L*' New Zealand 1992	206
Anthony Bland England 1992	207
Ward of Court Ireland 1995	214

Case of Karen Quinlan

In re Quinlan, 137 NJ Sup 227, 348 A2d 801, modified and remanded, 70 NJ 10, 355 A 2d 647 *cert denied*, 429 US 922 (1976).

Karen, aged 21 years, was found on 15 April 1975, unconscious in bed at the home of young friends after a session of alcohol and drugs. Two episodes of respiratory arrest lasting 15 minutes were recorded. After some 5 months on a respirator she remained in a vegetative state in intensive care. Her father eventually accepted the view of his wife and other children that *Karen* would never regain consciousness. All the family were devout

Roman Catholics and it was only after reassurance from his local priest that the respirator could be regarded as extraordinary treatment that Joseph Quinlan raised the question of taking *Karen* off the respirator. Her neurologist, only months out of training and himself a Catholic, objected strongly to this proposed course of action. Only a few months before, there had been a very sensational trial of an obstetrician who was convicted for having failed to do everything to save the life of a fetus, and this is believed to have influenced the doctors and their lawyers. Her father hired an idealistic young lawyer, Paul Armstrong, who was later to become famous for supporting other 'right to die' cases. The hospital tried to stop the case going to court, maintaining that it was physicians rather than the relatives who had the right to decide.

At the Superior Court of New Jersey in November 1975 her father sought to be appointed her *guardian ad litem* in place of the lawyer whom the court had appointed as her guardian as soon her father had indicated his wish to remove the respirator. That guardian declared in court that he had one simple role – to do every single thing to keep *Karen Quinlan* alive. The New Jersey Attorney General opposed the application because it would open the door to euthanasia. The neurologist's lawyer implored the judge not to impose a death sentence on *Karen*, maintaining that turning off the respirator would be like putting her in a gas chamber. These lawyers held that to withdraw treatment would be against the antieuthanasia policy of the AMA and the Catholic Church, and that it would not conform to medical standards and traditions. However, senior neurologists who appeared for the plaintiff emphasized that there was no prospect of recovery, and that it was accepted (if so far unspoken) medical practice to withdraw treatment in hopeless cases. The Quinlans maintained that *Karen* had twice said that she would not wish to be kept alive as a vegetable on machines. However, the judge decided that as these statements were remote and impersonal and were not written they lacked significant probative weight. The trial judge denied authorization of discontinuance of the life-supporting apparatus and refused to appoint *Karen*'s father as her guardian.

The Supreme Court of New Jersey heard an appeal in January 1976 and decided the case at the end of March 1976 – almost a year after *Karen* suffered brain damage. By this time, the New Jersey Catholic bishops had submitted an *amicus curiae* to the court arguing that a decision to withdraw extraordinary treatment would be morally correct, quoting the Pope's *allocutio* to anaesthetists in 1957 (see p. 98). In spite of this, a Vatican theologian criticized the Quinlans for requesting euthanasia (at the time of the trial but not in court). The Bishop of New Jersey assailed the Vatican bureaucrats and no more was heard from them. The unanimous judgement of the court noted that there was now no conflict between theology, medicine and the law on the issues in this case. The judges agreed that there was no clear evidence of *Karen*'s own views about what she would wish to be done. The justices expressed surprise at the importance that the physicians put on the distinction between withholding and withdrawing treatment, as they considered the differences between these and between omissions and acts to be rather flimsy. They declared that the State's interest in preserving life wanes in proportion to the prognosis for regaining awareness.

They considered that the case for withdrawing treatment rested on *Karen*'s constitutional right to privacy, and that this right could be exercised by her father. They considered that the decision to withdraw treatment should be made by the family and the physicians rather than a court, and that the trial judge had therefore been correct in not authorizing termination of life-supporting apparatus. However, he had been wrong to withhold letters of guardianship from the plaintiff (*Karen*'s father) and to have appointed a stranger in his stead. The Supreme Court decided unanimously that Joseph Quinlan should become *Karen*'s legal guardian, and that the respirator could be turned off at his request. If they complied with this request the hospital and the physicians would be granted legal immunity from charges of homicide or neglect. The court also suggested, but did not require, that a hospital ethics committee should resolve any further doubts that might arise.

In the event, the hospital was reluctant to follow the spirit of the court's decision. An administrator, who was a nun, declared that 'We don't kill people at this hospital', but she agreed to try to arrange transfer to a nursing home. As none of these would accept a patient on a respirator the physicians agreed to begin trying to wean her off the respirator. As this was gradually done it became clear that she was no longer dependent on this form of life support. The hospital now demanded that she should be sent to a nursing home but still there was none willing to take her. Only after Medicaid officials forced a public nursing home to take her was she transferred, in June 1976 6 months after the final court judgement. Although her parents agreed to a DNR order and that no antibiotics should be given for infections, she continued to be tube fed and she lived for ten more years, dying in June 1985.

In the same 1994 issue of the *New England Journal of Medicine* that the Multi-Society Task Force on the vegetative state was published there was a paper describing the detailed neuropathology of *Karen*'s brain and also an editorial titled 'After Quinlan: the dilemma of the persistent vegetative state' (1). The latter commentator noted that 'We owe Joseph and Julia Quinlan our gratitude for turning their personal calamity into a public benefit by launching the right-to-die movement'. She also added 'The Quinlans, with their characteristic openness and courage, close the chapter on their daughter's death by permitting the publication of the post-mortem examination of her brain'.

REFERENCES

1 Angell M. After Quinlan: the dilemma of the persistent vegetative state. *N Engl J Med* 1994; 330: 1524–5

Case of Clarence Herbert

Barber v. *Superior Court*, 195 Cal Rptr 484 (1983)

This court case bore the name of the physician (*Barber*) who was charged with murder, not the affected patient. Clarence Herbert was 55-years-old when he underwent abdominal surgery in August 1981. He had a cardiopulmonary collapse an hour after surgery after which a neurological opinion was that, because of severe brain damage, he had irreversible coma and his condition was hopeless. His wife, recalling her husband's comment before the operation 'If something goes wrong, don't let the doctors keep me alive', requested removal of all life-support machines. A written version of this request was signed by the patient's wife and children and witnessed by two nurses. *Dr Barber*, a senior internist in charge of intensive care, agreed with Dr Nedjl, the surgeon, that the respirator should be disconnected. As the patient was still alive 2 days later the family requested that no medication be given and that 'everything be pulled out'. The intravenous fluid line was disconnected and a nasogastric tube was also removed, and he died 6 days later. Although referred to in some later reports as having been vegetative, it is clear that he did not fit that diagnosis – though that might well have been the outcome had he been allowed to survive longer.

It seems that only 5 days before Mr Herbert's operation the hospital had circulated a memorandum recommending that a decision to 'pull the plug' should not be made without consultation with legal counsel. However, one journalist's report asserts that Drs *Barber* and Nedjl decided that to seek legal advice in this case would only hold things up and drive a wedge between the physicians and the family – whose wishes were very clear and in writing. After disconnecting the respirator, there was some conflict between Dr Nedjl and Sandra Bardinilla, a nursing supervisor, regarding continuing with a humidifier to avoid thickening of secretions in the lumen of the endotracheal tube. It seems that she also had doubts about the wisdom of withdrawing treatment. She copied the patient's medical records and took her grievances to her supervisors and others in the hospital hierarchy. Getting no support she took her information to the Los Angeles County Department of Health Services – an agency charged with supervising health-care providers. After an investigation, this body called the District Attorney's office and a resolute deputy DA filed a murder charge against the two doctors when it was already a year since Herbert's death.

In March 1983, a Municipal Court judge dismissed the charges at a preliminary hearing, finding no evidence of malicious intent because the doctors had acted under the reasonable belief that the patient had irreversible coma and their actions also had the consent of the family. There was no evidence of conspiracy by these two physicians to cover up malpractice that might have led to his hopeless condition, as was alleged by the prosecutors as a possible motive. The judge did not accept the claim that food and water artificially given were basic care rather than medical treatment (1). The DA appealed and in May 1983 a Superior Court judge reinstated the charges. The main reason was, apparently, concern that it had not been sufficiently well established that Herbert's condition was irreversible, as the court had conflicting medical evidence about the chances of some recovery after such a brief period in coma. Court cases about withdrawal of ANH from patients in a vegetative state have certainly all been for patients who had been in that state for long periods. However, for acutely ill patients in intensive care units it had by then become commonplace to withdraw life-sustaining treatment after only days if the prognosis was considered hopeless.

In October 1983, the California Court of Appeal dismissed the murder charge without the physicians going to trial, and this decision was not appealed. The court echoed much of what had been stated by the President's Commission (published earlier that year) about limiting the use of life-prolonging treatment for the hopelessly ill. According to this court, medical treatment had to be used only if it would benefit the patient, and it declared that feeding was to be equated with other forms of medical treatment – the first appellate court so to decide. It proposed a best interests test for whether treatment was appropriate, including such factors as relief from suffering, the restoration of functioning, the quality as well as the expected extent of the life sustained and the impact of the decision on the family. There was no duty to provide life-sustaining treatment once it had become futile in the opinion of qualified medical personnel. It held that a physician who acted within established professional standards would incur no legal liability. In this respect this court gave a greater decision-making role to the physician than later courts were to do. None the less it stated that the family was the proper surrogate and that there was no need for such a surrogate to seek prior judicial approval. This remains the only occasion on which physicians have been charged with a criminal or civil offence after withdrawing treatment from a patient deemed hopelessly ill.

REFERENCES

1 Paris JJ, Reardon FE. Court responses to withholding or withdrawing artificial nutrition and fluids. *JAMA* 1985; 253: 2243–5

Case of Claire Conroy

In the matter of Claire Conroy, 98 N.J. 321 (1985)

Claire Conroy was an 85-year-old nursing-home resident whose only relative was a nephew who had been her legal guardian for several years. She had hypertension, heart disease and diabetes and had advanced organic dementia. Although occasionally groaning or smiling she was essentially unaware but she was not regarded as vegetative; she would now probably be considered in a minimally conscious state. Her nephew, who visited each week and had earlier opposed efforts to end life support, asked in 1983 for her nasogastric tube to be removed, but the physicians would not comply. The trial court ruled in favour of the nephew but she died 13 days later with the tube still in place. After her death an intermediate appellate court reversed this ruling. Although any decision about treatment was no longer relevant, the Supreme Court of New Jersey heard an appeal more than a year after her death, with the decision coming many months later in January 1985. It decided that it would not have granted the nephew's request, but in explaining the reasons for this the court effectively made recommendations for dealing with such patients in nursing homes.

It defined such patients as those with serious and permanent mental and physical impairment, unlikely ever to gain competence and who would probably die within one year. It rejected the appellate opinion that to discontinue life support in patients not irreversibly comatose or vegetative would be active euthanasia, and declared that in some circumstances it would be proper to withdraw nasogastric feeding and other life support. It would authorize this if it was clear that the patient would have refused or if administering it would be considered to be inhumane.

The court went on to define how a decision might be made. Evidence for a subjective test for the patient's wishes would include a written living will, a previous oral directive, a durable power of attorney or an appointed proxy. In the absence of these, the court would exercise its *parens patriae* power to act in the best interests of an incompetent person by allowing ANH to be withdrawn if it was disproportionately burdensome or contrary to the patient's values or interests. It would decide on the basis of either a limited or pure objective standard. The first would apply when there was only *some* trustworthy evidence that the patient would have refused treatment (casual comments or the patient's general values). In that event there would need to be evidence of unavoidable pain as part of the burden of continuing treatment. For the purely objective standard (a best interests judgment) there would have to be stricter evidence of an unbearable life, including pain – thereby making treatment inhumane. The court rejected any quality of life judgement other than extreme pain. The one dissenting justice (of six) did not support this need for pain to justify withdrawing treatment. He wrote: 'The exclusive pain criterion denies relief to a class of people who, at the very end of life, might strongly disapprove of an artificially extended existence in spite of the absence of pain'. The court made no reference to involving ethics committees as recommended by the same court in *Quinlan* – perhaps because such committees do not usually operate in nursing homes. Instead it suggested using the State Ombudsman, a facility available for nursing home-patients in New Jersey.

This was a landmark case in several respects (1,2). It was the first time that tube feeding was accepted as medical treatment that could be withdrawn from a chronically ill patient (the *Barber* case dealt with intravenous feeding in an acute situation). It was also the first to indicate that this might be withdrawn from a patient not in a vegetative state. Its comments on pain clearly had no application to vegetative patients and subsequent courts have not accepted pain as a necessary condition for declaring that a given treatment be disproportionately burdensome.

REFERENCES

1 Curran WJ. Defining appropriate medical care in providing nutrients for the dying. *N Engl J Med* 1985; 313: 940–2
2 Paris JJ, Reardon FE. Court responses to withholding or withdrawing artificial nutrition and fluids. *JAMA* 1985; 253: 2243–5

Case of Paul Brophy

Brophy v. *New England Sinai Hospital,* 497 NE 2d 626 (Sup Jud Ct Mass 1986)

Paul Brophy was a 47-year-old former fireman and emergency medical technician who suffered haemorrhage from a basilar artery aneurysm in March 1983 and after surgery was left in a vegetative state. In July 1983, his family requested a DNR order and in December 1983 a gastrostomy tube was inserted. In February 1985, when he had been vegetative for almost 2 years, his wife (a nurse) who was his legal guardian asked for feeding to be discontinued in accordance with her husband's previously expressed wishes. His Catholic family of seven brothers and sisters, his mother and five adult children all supported this. His wishes had been made clear on several occasions. At the time of *Quinlan* he had said he did not ever want to be on a life-support system. Some 5 years previously, after he had rescued a man who died of severe burns some weeks later, he had said that it would have been better if they had been a bit later and the victim had died in the fire. He then told his brother, 'If I'm ever like that, just pull the plug'. After yet another rescue, of a teenage pedestrian who lived 2–3 days on life support, *Brophy* told his wife 'No way, don't ever let that happen to me'.

On the day the case was filed, the Probate judge appointed a lawyer as *guardian ad litem*. He also ordered that the long-standing DNR order and the nonaggressive treatment order be set aside. The Board of Directors of the hospital had already voted that if the court did order them to stop feeding they would refuse to comply and would appeal. After the *guardian ad litem* had reported back, arguing against removal of the tube, there was a hearing. The judge accepted that there was clear evidence that *Brophy* would have refused tube feeding if he could and that the family agreed with this. However, having heard conflicting medical and theological viewpoints the judge decided that there was no evidence that continuing tube feeding was burdensome and that while the placing of the tube might have been termed invasive the current treatment was not. Stopping feeding was not, therefore, intended to relieve burdens but to cause his death, which was not otherwise imminent. As such it could be construed as euthanasia. He considered that the state's interest in the preservation of life outweighed the prior wishes of the patient because the treatment was not burdensome. Nor was *Brophy* able to suffer mental anguish from his present condition. The judge was also impressed by the evidence led by those opposing the application about the cruel and violent death that would result from dehydration, while accepting that *Brophy* would probably not feel pain. The judge therefore agreed that the hospital could continue with tube feeding, but ruled that the orders about DNR and nonaggressive treatment should be reinstated.

The Supreme Judicial Court of Massachusetts heard an appeal in May 1986 and gave judgement in September 1986. In addition to the original evidence this court received no less than six *amici curiae* from various bodies, all but one pleading that withdrawal of feeding be allowed. Three of these five were from medical societies, one from the Society for Right to Die and the other the Civil Liberties Union. The appeal judgement referred to several previous court cases where treatment withdrawal had been permitted and also to the President's Commission. It concluded that the state's interest in the preservation of life did not overcome *Brophy*'s right to refuse treatment. To maintain that such treatment was ordinary was to ignore the total circumstances of *Brophy*'s situation. Because this treatment could lead to his life being sustained in this condition for many years this treatment should be considered not only intrusive but extraordinary. It agreed with the *Conroy* court that the focus should be on the patient's desires, not on the type of treatment. In any event, such withdrawal would be in accord with widely accepted medical practice, and death would be from natural causes. The conclusion was that the present hospital need not be forced to withdraw treatment but it was ordered to assist the guardian (his wife) to secure a transfer to another institution. The guardian was then authorized to order such measures as she might deem necessary and appropriate.

This was a four to three decision. One justice dissented from the whole judgement. He maintained that to regard food and water as medical treatment was an outrageously erroneous premise. He considered that the court had endorsed euthanasia and suicide. He regarded the decision as a triumph for the forces of secular humanism which he regarded as modern paganism. Two others dissented in part. Whilst agreeing with much of the judgement, one felt that not enough notice was taken of the risk of seeming to condone suicide and euthanasia, or of defending the sanctity of life. He was suspicious of substituted judgment being equated with actual judgement, and that to do so could be regarded as paternalism masquerading as autonomy. The other maintained that *Brophy*'s wish not to be treated was because of a quality of life judgement, not the wish to be free of burdens. The court's decision would be more acceptable if the patient had been terminally ill as in some previous court cases.

In accordance with the court order, *Brophy* was transferred to another hospital. The US Supreme Court declined to hear the case when emergency petitions were made and *Brophy* died after withdrawal of ANH, about 6 weeks after the judgement. He thus became the first living person for whom a court had sanctioned withdrawal of ANH and who had died as a result of the court's decision (1).

REFERENCES

1 Beresford HR. The Brophy case: whose life is it? *Neurology* 1981; 37: 1357–8

Case of Mary O'Connor

In re O'Connor, 72 N.Y. 2d 517, 531 N.E. 2d 607, 534 N.Y.S. 2d 886 (1988)

Mary O'Connor was a 77-year-old widow who had had a series of strokes which left her suffering from multi-infarct dementia. In June 1988, she developed sepsis, pneumonia and dehydration and was transferred from a nursing home to hospital where she was treated with antibiotics and intravenous fluids. She was said to be able sometimes to answer simple questions and to obey commands. As she had become dehydrated when being hand fed in the nursing home, the hospital wished to use a nasogastric feeding tube. Her two daughters, both nurses, refused permission, believing that their mother would not have wanted any form of life support. They claimed that their mother had frequently said that she would not want artificial life support, considering it monstrous to keep people alive by such means. She had said that she would not want to go on living if she could not take care of herself and make her own decisions. However, she had not specifically mentioned feeding tubes. It was known that she had worked in hospitals for two decades, and witnessing her husband and two brothers dying of cancer was also believed to have influenced her views on life-prolonging treatment.

The hospital ethics committee considered that feeding should not be withheld and the hospital in July 1988 sought court authorization to insert a feeding tube. The trial and appellate courts refused the hospital permission to institute artificial feeding against the family's wishes but, pending a further appeal, her nutrition was maintained by intravenous feeding. In October 1988, the New York Court of Appeals reversed those rulings in a four to three decision. It argued that treatment should be withheld only if there was clear and convincing evidence that the patient did not want certain procedures to be employed under specified circumstances. It dismissed her previous statements as immediate reactions to unsettling experiences and cautioned in general that any patient's previous statements might not indicate reflection and resolve. New York did not at that time have a living will statute but this court did acknowledge that if this person's wishes had been in writing it would have suggested her seriousness of purpose. The court opined that this would have avoided its being asked to make a life-or-death decision based upon casual remarks. It also rejected treatment decisions based on assessments of the best interests of an incompetent patient.

In rejecting the legitimacy of a family's evidence about a patient's informally expressed wishes and in refusing to allow a decision based on best interests, the New York court was going against the trend set by many previous courts (1,2). Since *Quinlan* there had by then been 16 vegetative cases and one of dementia in 12 different state courts allowing abatement of treatment, nine of them involving withholding or withdrawing tube feeding.

No doubt reflecting the fact that this patient was not vegetative, the appeal court raised two other issues. One was that the patient might improve, although two physicians had testified originally that no improvement was expected. It was 3 months since that prediction, but the appeal court could hear no new evidence (i.e. that no improvement had occurred in that period) – it could only debate the decisions made on the original evidence. The other issue was that because she had some residual consciousness she might suffer if feeding was denied. This ignored that it was already good medical practice to provide drugs to deal with symptoms during withdrawal of, for example, mechanical ventilation at a patient's request. In the event *O'Connor* did not improve and she died in August 1989 with the tube still in place – 10 months after the final court case had authorized its placement.

REFERENCES

1 Gasner MR. *Cruzan* v. *Harmon* and in the matter of *O'Connor*. *JAGS* 1990; 38: 594–9
2 Lo B, Rouse F, Dornbrand L. Family decision-making on trial. Who decides for incompetent patients? *N Engl J Med* 1990; 322: 128–32

Case of Nancy Cruzan

Cruzan v. *Harmon,* 760 S.W. 2d 408 (Mo. 1988)
Cruzan v. *Director, Missouri Dept of Health,* 110 S. Ct. 2841 (1990)

In 1983, at the age of 25 years, *Nancy Cruzan* sustained a severe head injury and was left in a vegetative state with a gastrostomy tube for feeding. In 1986, her parents contacted the Society for the Right to Die about their right to request withdrawal of tube feeding. As the hospital was unwilling to comply with this they decided to take the case to court. In 1987, they secured an order that they become her legal guardians. In July 1988, a trial court heard *Nancy* described as a vivacious outgoing person who took pride in her appearance. It heard from her housemate that *Nancy* had told her, in reaction to the death of this housemate's sister a year before her own accident, that 'she didn't want to live as a vegetable'. This witness added that she was sure that if *Nancy* could not do for herself even halfway, let alone not at all, she would not want to live that way; and that *Nancy* hoped that her family would know that. The family, who visited her regularly, maintained that *Nancy* would not want to continue living in her present condition. The court ruled that tube feedings could be removed but the Attorney General for Missouri (Harmon) appealed the decision.

In November 1988, the Missouri Supreme Court reversed the lower court in a four to three decision. It did so in spite of having itself cited over 50 cases from 16 other states where treatment withdrawal had been allowed, and in the words of one dissenting judge 'of having failed to point to a single case in support of its final conclusion'. It maintained that families could not forgo treatments without the most rigid of formalities – a living will or clear and convincing evidence of the patient's refusal to be treated. It found that there was no reliable evidence that *Nancy* would have refused artificial feeding and went on to express scepticism about all living wills. (Yet Missouri had a living will statute at that time, although refusal of nutrition was not allowed as a treatment preference.) Accepting that her parents had the highest motives the court considered that it had to decide for other patients not as blessed as *Nancy* in this regard. It declared that tube feedings were not burdensome or heroically invasive – the invasion had been when the tube was inserted. Although not deliberating on whether or not artificial feeding was medical treatment, the court did state that 'common sense tells us that food and water do not treat an illness, they maintain a life'. This led to the main reason for the decision – that the State had an unqualified interest in the preservation of life that outweighed any consideration of the quality of that life or of any constitutional or common-law rights to have treatment withheld. The state made clear that it would meet the $130 000 annual costs of medical and nursing care for as long as her life was sustained.

The US Supreme Court heard evidence in December 1989. As well as evidence from the involved parties, it also received a number of *amici curiae* including those from the Society for the Right to Die and from the American Geriatric Society both of which argued for treatment withdrawal and for allowing family surrogates to make such a decision. *Amici curiae* were received also from the Association of Retarded Citizens and others representing vulnerable persons, whose life and well-being would, they claimed, be jeopardized if the Missouri ruling were reversed. On the day of the court hearing there was an extended discussion program on public service television, with doctors, lawyers and ethicists arguing the case. In February 1990, a national public opinion poll reported that of 805 respondents 88% voted in favour of families deciding about treatment for an incompetent patient who had left no instructions, 8% that physicians should decide and 1% that courts should (1). A few weeks before the judgement in June 1990 there were papers in the *New England Journal of Medicine* urging the court to find in favour of the family (2,3).

The five to four decision reaffirmed that competent patients had a constitutional right to refuse unwanted treatment. Unlike many previous courts, it saw this as based on the right of liberty rather than on the right of privacy or the common law right of self-determination. In regard to the problem of incompetent patients exercising that right the main question before the court was whether Missouri could set its own standards in deciding about such cases. The Supreme Court decided that a state had a constitutional right to do so – reflecting the Supreme Court's reluctance in most issues to interfere with state laws. It stated that not only could Missouri require clear and convincing evidence of the patient's own views, but it could claim an unqualified interest in the preservation of life, could exclude quality of life as a determining factor and could err on the side of continuing treatment. However, it went on to declare that no other states need decide similarly. It decided that the constitution allowed the states to rely on families to make decisions but did not mandate this. It noted, however, that there was no automatic assurance that family views would always accurately reflect those of the patient. In a concurring opinion one justice emphasized that artificial feeding could not be distinguished from other forms of medical treatment. She also wrote strongly in support of advance directives and added that states might consider as an equally probative source of evidence (of the patient's wishes) her appointment of a proxy to make health-care decisions on her behalf. She also noted that the court's decision did not preclude a future determination that the Constitution might require all states to implement the decisions of a duly appointed surrogate.

For three of the dissenting justices it was declared that there was a fundamental constitutional right to refuse treatment rather than simply a liberty interest. (Such a fundamental right would be less susceptible to the vagaries of legal regulations imposed by different states.) To emphasize this they stated that no state interest should outweigh the right of a patient to refuse treatment. They asserted that the Missouri restriction would probably lead to more deaths than current practice because, if withdrawing unsuccessful treatment was to be made so difficult, doctors might become reluctant to initiate trials of therapy that might be of benefit. They considered that the improperly biased procedural obstacles imposed by Missouri impermissibly burdened the right to refuse treatment by making it less likely that *Nancy Cruzan*'s wishes could be accurately determined. It was families or designated surrogates who should make these kinds of decision. They argued that the Missouri rules were out of touch with reality, because most people do not write elaborate documents about their future treatment. In effect, they maintained that the Missouri procedure would transform incompetent human beings into passive subjects of medical technology. The remaining dissenter maintained that the constitution required that the best interests of patients be respected, and that the state may not override the wishes or best interests of a patient.

Although the majority decision appeared to support the position of Missouri, that State did not, in the event, press its advantage when a few months later the Cruzan family petitioned the original trial court to rehear their request to discontinue tube feeding, because new witnesses had come forward. Indeed, the State of Missouri requested and was granted permission to withdraw from the case. *Nancy*'s attending physician declared that he too had changed his mind and was now in favour of stopping feeding. The family's petition was therefore not opposed. The new witnesses were two women who had worked with *Nancy* at a school for deaf and blind children in 1978 (5 years before her accident). They testified that she had said then that if she were a vegetable she would not want to be fed by force or kept alive by machines. In December, the same judge who had heard the first court case accepted that there was now clear and convincing evidence of *Nancy*'s intent and he ruled for a second time that tube feeding could be stopped. This was done soon after the ruling, when injunctions to stop withdrawal had been denied by both state and federal courts, and in spite of demonstrations from pro-life protestors and offers from some other institutions to take over her care and to maintain feeding. She died in late December 1990, aged 33, after almost 8 years in a vegetative state. Some 6 months later her father formed the Nancy Cruzan Foundation for which he then worked. Its aims were to support families in similar situations, to encourage the use of advance directives and to work with the medical profession to deal better with families. In 1991, Joe Cruzan received a humanitarian award for helping to further quality in medicine. However, 5 years after this, at the age of 62, he committed suicide.

This case attracted unprecedented publicity, with the New York Times of

26 June devoting a whole page to long extracts of the opinions of concurring and dissenting justices, as well as columns of comment. There soon followed a number of commentaries in medical journals anxious to interpret the consequences of the *Cruzan* decision for medical practice. There was concern that misinterpretation might lead to serious adverse consequences for hopelessly ill patients, their families and health-care professionals. More reflective comments continued for several years. The most terse immediate response was a single column statement in the *New England Journal of Medicine* from 34 bioethicists (made up of seven physicians, six lawyers, a nurse and 20 philosophers). Its five points were summarized in the fifth – 'The *Cruzan* decision does not alter the laws, ethical standards, or clinical practices permitting the forgoing of life-sustaining treatment that have evolved in the United States since the *Quinlan* case' (4).

In a longer commentary in the same issue of the same journal a jurist qualified in public health agreed with the bioethicists but was less optimistic about there being no change in practice as a result of this case (5). He considered that the court had ceded incredible leeway to the states, so that no one was now safe in those states that wished to control the health-care decisions and deaths of its citizens. However, he welcomed the agreement that artificial feeding should be regarded as medical treatment because this could mean that state statutes that treat tube feeding as different from other life-sustaining treatments might now be declared unconstitutional. That the court had ignored physicians (having included them in the general reference to 'hospital employees') betrayed, he believed, a complete lack of attention to medical reality. Lawyers certainly would not ignore physicians and indeed were likely now to deluge them with conflicting opinions and demands in the wake of the *Cruzan* decision.

The formal AMA response again emphasized that nothing had really been changed by the *Cruzan* decision (6). Indeed it considered that it had enlarged the right to refuse treatment in many respects. It pointed out how few of the 130 cases that had gone to court for limiting life-sustaining treatment had resulted in the family's conclusion about the wishes or best interests of the patient being challenged. Also, that no person had ever been found legally liable for withdrawing life-sustaining treatment without court permission. It stressed the need for physicians to initiate discussions with their patients about life-sustaining treatment and to encourage them to write an advance directive, in order to minimize uncertainty if and when a decision had to be made when they had become incompetent. As a spur to this, the Patient Self-Determination Act was enacted within months of the *Cruzan* decision and became law in November 1991. This requires hospitals and nursing homes to give patients on admission written information about their right to refuse treatment and to make an advance directive.

Further reviews by medical ethicists largely echoed these initial opinions (7) but one discussed what evidence of a patient's wishes might be construed as clear and convincing (8). This had been described in the *O'Connor* court as 'truth sufficient to persuade a judge and jury that the patient held a firm and settled commitment to the termination of life support'. It required more certainty than 'preponderance of the evidence' (more likely than not) but less than 'beyond reasonable doubt'. Although all agreed that written directives provided the best evidence, many courts had accepted oral evidence – though without always pronouncing the mantra of 'clear and convincing'. This commentary also explicitly listed some potentially harmful consequences of the *Cruzan* decision. These were undermining the role of the family, promoting defensive medicine that might result in continuing with nonbeneficial and unwanted treatment as the safest option, and encouraging cynicism and disregard of the law by physicians.

It seems, in practice, that the main effect of *Cruzan* was to clarify what had already become good practice without resulting in the constraints on compassionate joint decision making by physicians and families that some had feared (9). *Cruzan* prompted an increased interest in advance directives and many statutes dealing with these were modified after that case to allow refusals for vegetative as well as terminally ill patients, and specifically to allow withdrawal of ANH.

REFERENCES

Before the Supreme Court decision
1 Coyle M. How Americans view high court. *Natl Law J* 1990; 26 Feb
2 Angell M. Prisoners of technology: the case of *Nancy Cruzan*. *N Engl J Med* 1990; 322: 1226–8
3 Lo B, Rouse F, Dornbrand L. Family decision on trial; who decides for incompetent patients? *N Engl J Med* 1990; 322: 1228–32

After the Supreme Court decision

4 Annas G, Arnold B, Aroskar M et al. Bioethicists' statement on the US Supreme Court's *Cruzan* decision. *N Engl J Med* 1990; 323: 686–7

5 Annas G. *Nancy Cruzan* and the right to die. *N Engl J Med* 1990; 323: 670–73

6 Orentlicher D (for the General Council of the AMA). The right to die after *Cruzan*. *JAMA* 1990; 264: 2444–6

7 White BD, Siegler M, Singer PA et al. What does *Cruzan* mean to the practising physician? *Arch Intern Med* 1991; 151: 925–8

8 Lo B, Steinbrook R. Beyond the *Cruzan* case; the US Supreme Court and medical practice. *Ann Intern Med* 1991; 114: 895–901

9 Beresford HR. The persistent vegetative state: a view across the legal divide. *Ann N Y Acad Sci* 1997; 835: 386–94

Case of Frederick Cyril Clarke

Clarke v. *Hurst* Supreme Court of South Africa (Durban and Coast Local Division) July 1992

This man suffered a cardiac arrest during a medical procedure when aged 64 years and was left in a vegetative state. He remained in hospital with a nasogastric feeding tube for the next 4 years. His wife then applied to the court to appoint her as *curatrix personae* with powers to withhold agreement to medical treatment and to authorize the discontinuation of nasogastric or other non-natural feeding. She was anxious to see that her husband's previously expressed wishes were respected. He was a doctor with administrative responsibility for the hospitals in his region and he was a member of the South African Voluntary Euthanasia Society. He had enacted a living will stating that he did not wish to kept alive by artificial means or heroic measures if there was no reasonable expectation of recovery from extreme physical or mental disability. His four children and his two sisters supported his wife. The court-appointed *curator ad litem* did not oppose the application but the Attorney General for the Province did. He considered that the court should not tie his hands by preventing him from pursuing a criminal prosecution if the application were granted.

The judge ruled that despite the opposition of the Attorney General the Court could in an appropriate case declare that a certain course of future conduct would not constitute a crime. He said that the emotionally involved wife had the right to have her legal position determined by the court after it had viewed the evidence dispassionately and objectively. It was accepted that a competent patient could refuse even life-sustaining treatment. The judge ruled that it followed that, where a person while in sound mind had directed that he should be allowed to die in certain circumstances, there was no reason why a curator should not have power to give effect to that person's directions. However, he pointed out that the curator was not a mere agent to give effect to prior directions from the patient, but had a duty to assess the patient's best interests, which might not always correspond with his wishes. He went on to quote with approval the judgements in four cases in the Supreme Court of New Jersey, including *Quinlan*, but warned that they did not provide an answer to the interface with the criminal law in South Africa. In considering the justification for conduct that would otherwise be unlawful the grounds had become stereotyped and did not embrace this new type of situation. The law was but a translation of society's fundamental values into policies. The question was whether discontinuing treatment would be wrongful as judged by the legal convictions and *boni mores* of our society. Reasonableness rather than logic dictated the formation of society's legal and moral convictions about what was right and wrong. The decision depended on the quality of life that would remain for the patient. Decisions to allow terminally ill patients to die were taken regularly by doctors. Advances in medicine required a change in society's attitude to the process of dying, and decisions about life-sustaining procedures involved a balancing exercise. In addition to the American cases, reference was made to *Re J* and *Re B*, handicapped infants dealt with by the English courts, as evidence that it was reasonable to assess a person's quality of life when making such a decision.

The judge declared that artificial feeding had no symbolic significance for the patient who was unaware. In determining legal liability he did not think there was any distinction between withholding and withdrawing treatment. The mere restoration of certain biological functions could not be regarded as the saving of a patient's life, and such unsuccessful treatment should be discontinued. Judged by society's legal convictions, the feeding of this patient did not serve the purpose of supporting human life as it was commonly known, and it would therefore be reasonable to discontinue it. The action would be in the best interests of the patient. The cause of death would be the original brain damage. The court should guard against allowing liability to exceed the bounds of reasonableness, fairness and justice. The application was granted.

Case of L

Auckland Health Board v. *Attorney-General* (Re L) [1993] 1 NZLR 235

This 59-year-old man had developed severe Guillain–Barre syndrome which had gradually paralysed all the muscles in his body. For the last year he had been dependent on a ventilator and unable to interact in any way with his surroundings. He displayed no awareness and it was uncertain whether he could see or hear. He was described as being both locked in and locked out by reason of his total paralysis. With the approval of the ethics committee of the hospital and of the patient's wife, the hospital and the treating doctor sought a declaration from the court that it would not be unlawful to withdraw ventilation. The Attorney General opposed this because it would impinge upon the prosecutorial discretion and preroga- tive powers of the Crown (to institute criminal proceedings). He was also concerned that the court would be entering upon a domain that should properly be left to members of the medical profession. It would be better, he said, for the courts to offer guidelines to allow doctors to proceed without unwieldy applications to the courts – which were undesirable because they were cumbersome and imposed an extreme burden on the relatives of the patient. In making a declaratory order in this case in August 1992, the judge expressed the diffident hope that it would assist and encourage doctors to reach these critical decisions in future without recourse to the courts. But the doctors' request for guidance as to the lawfulness of their proposed actions in this case had been wholly reason- able.

He accepted that the sanctity of life was not absolute and that competent patients were entitled to refuse the initiation or continuation of life- sustaining treatment. He referred to the case of *Nancy B* who also had severe Guillain–Barre, but had been competent to request the removal of her respirator, which the Quebec Superior Court had allowed (1). The judge observed that, with the use of life-support systems, it could become unclear whether life was being sustained or death being deferred. Whether a body was devoid of mind or, as in the case of *Mr L*, a brain destitute of a body, did not matter in any sensible way. Either way they lacked self- awareness or awareness of the surroundings in any cognitive sense. The issue of treatment withdrawal in these circumstances was essentially a medical one which could not be resolved by strict logic, and certainly not by legal logic. It was best determined by common principles of humanity and common sense. Doctors had a lawful excuse to discontinue ventilation when there was no medical justification for continuing it. To require treatment that served only to defer the death of the patient was to confound the purpose of medicine. The continuation of ventilation might be lawful, but that did not make it unlawful to discontinue it if this accorded with good medical practice.

He then referred to *Re J*, where an English court had ruled that a doctor was not under a duty to prolong life if this was not in his judgement in the best interests of the patient. Nothing in the inherent purpose of recent scientific advances could require doctors to treat the dying as if they were curable. It was crucial for the patient, and also in the overall interests of society, that when doctors are exercising their best judgement they should not be inhibited by their own self-interest in avoiding criminal sanctions. He then referred to a number of other court cases from which it was clear that doctors could not be held legally responsible for the death of a patient after the appropriate withdrawal of life-support systems. Nor was the doctor factually the agent of death when this was due to allowing death from the original disease that had been arrested for a time. It was surely never intended that medical science and technology be used to prolong the biological life of patients bereft of the prospect of returning to even a limited exercise of human life. The declaration granted stated that withdrawal of ventilation would not constitute culpable homicide.

REFERENCES

1 *Nancy B* v. *Hotel-Dieu de Quebec* [1992] 86 DLR (4th) 385

Case of Anthony Bland

Airedale NHS Trust v. *Bland* [1993] 1 All ER 821

In April 1989, Anthony Bland, then 17 years old, suffered anoxic brain damage when his chest was crushed in a football stadium disaster where over 90 spectators died and at least one other victim was left in a vegetative state. After initial treatment in Sheffield he was transferred to a hospital nearer his home where he was fortunate to be under the care of a general

physician who had also trained as a neurologist. He received active rehabilitation but after 4 months he was still in a vegetative state and his parents
raised the matter of discontinuing tube feeding to let him die. His doctor
was sympathetic to this request but felt it wise to consult the Sheffield
coroner – who would have to hold an inquest into his death, as this would
clearly not be from natural causes. This coroner was both medically and
legally qualified and he wrote that if his death followed the withdrawal of
life-sustaining treatment he would feel bound to initiate criminal proceedings. He advised that legal opinion at a higher level should be sought. In the
event, it was over 3 years before the case reached the highest courts in the
land. In the interim there was considerable interest in the print press and
this led to TV documentaries about the case, and it emerged that legal
advice to doctors about a similar case in Scotland had been much more
relaxed (p. 148). This led some to suggest that one solution would be to
transfer *Bland* to Scotland.

The case reached the Family Division of the High Court when the
hospital Trust applied for a declaration that withdrawal of ANH would not
be unlawful. Five medical witnesses agreed that *Bland* was in a permanent
vegetative state and that continuing treatment was not in his best interests.
Only one held that ANH was not medical treatment and should not be
withdrawn. The patient's father told the court that he was sure his son
would have refused continued treatment if he could, but he had never
expressed a view on this.

Counsel for the Trust argued that an incompetent patient should not be
disadvantaged by being unable to have treatment that he would probably
have refused withdrawn. Nor should health professionals be at legal risk if
acting in what they regarded as their patient's best interests, and in accord
with good medical practice. Other English courts had recently allowed
doctors to withhold life-saving treatment from severely handicapped infants who were not yet terminally ill. Counsel for the Attorney General,
who appeared at the court's request as *amicus curiae* because of the public
policy significance of the case, argued against an absolutist position in
matters such as this. To ignore quality of life was to show lack of respect for
the quality of life. He referred at length to *Cruzan* and to the decisions
about handicapped infants. He supported the application. It was opposed
by counsel for the Official Solicitor, a government legal office that acts as
guardian ad litem for minors and incompetent adults. He argued that ANH
was not medical treatment but basic care, and that reference to pain and

suffering in the infant cases was irrelevant as all the doctors had agreed that *Bland* was unconscious. If this application was granted it might begin a slippery slope to more decisions to deny treatment for vulnerable patients. Finally he equated withdrawal of ANH with cutting a climber's rope or a diver's air tube – which would be murder.

In his judgement, Sir Stephen Brown, President of the Family Division, ruled that ANH was medical treatment and that the cause of death after its withdrawal would be the initial brain damage. Withdrawal would be in accord with good medical practice as stated in the recent BMA document, and with decisions in other common law jurisdictions. Although he accepted that doctors could decide about best interests of their patients and about the appropriateness of withdrawing treatment he recommended that future cases should be brought to court for prior approval, with two medical opinions. This would be a safeguard for the doctors and would reassure the public.

Recognizing the significance of this landmark case both parties had agreed that whatever the court decided it would be appealed to secure a more authoritative ruling. The Official Solicitor duly appealed and less than three weeks later three appellate judges unanimously dismissed the appeal. Each judge wrote an opinion, and these revealed some differences in emphasis.

Sir Thomas Bingham, Master of the Rolls, began by observing that this case was not about euthanasia, nor with putting down the old and infirm, the mentally defective or the physically imperfect. He listed the principles of respect for the sanctity of life, the need for consent for medical treatment and that doctors must comply with instructions from a competent adult even if these appear to be irrational – and this applied even if the patient was incompetent when the time came. It followed that if *Bland* had left instructions to withhold treatment his doctors could lawfully have complied with these. Whether or not tube feeding was medical treatment it was certainly part of medical care. He doubted if it had ever been an object of medical care merely to prolong the life of an insensate patient with no hope of recovery.

He went on to note that several other jurisdictions had squarely confronted the issue of withdrawing treatment. Decisions in the courts in the US (Chapter 9), South Africa (p. 204) and New Zealand (p. 206), as well as a statement from the Law Commission of Canada (p. 183) all indicated that a presumption in favour of prolonging life was not irrebuttable.

English courts had already sanctioned the withholding of life-prolonging treatment from some severely handicapped infants (*Re C* and *Re J*) (1,2). He considered that best interests should take account of wider, less tangible, considerations than pain and suffering. Although assessment of best interests was a matter for doctors, the sanction of a court could be invoked to exclude medical error and to review divisions of opinion or conflicts of interest. He considered that while it seemed desirable that future cases of this kind should come to court it might be that with the passage of time a body of experience and practice would build up which would obviate the need for this in every case. As for the arguments of counsel for the Official Solicitor that withdrawing ANH would be like cutting a mountaineer's rope or a diver's air tube and would therefore be murder, Sir Thomas said that he did not accept any ingredient of this submission. In accepting the submissions for the hospital and the Attorney General he commented that he could not conceive what benefit *Bland's* continued existence could be thought to give him.

Lord Justice Butler-Sloss noted that best interests was more in line with English law than substituted judgement, and she warned that the views of the family should be treated with caution as they might have hidden motives. It was the duty of doctors to treat patients in their best interests, in accordance with a responsible and competent body of relevant professional opinion. Previous courts had rejected an absolutist approach to sanctity of life. To limit quality of life to the absence of extreme pain was to take a demeaning view of a human being. She was dismayed by the argument for the Official Solicitor that cardiac arrest or renal failure in a vegetative patient would justify major medical interventions. Such useless treatment was contrary to good medical practice and an affront to the patient's right to be respected. The reality of *Bland's* existence outweighed the abstract requirement to preserve life. Noting that the Mental Health Act of 1993 had included nursing within the ambit of medical treatment, she thought that medical care was a more inclusive term that would include tube feeding. To withdraw it would place the patient as he would have been before tube feeding was begun.

Lord Justice Hoffmann noted that in other situations we deny sanctity of life as an overriding principle – when allowing refusal of treatment and when not force-feeding prisoners. We had to reassure people that the law had full respect for life but that it did not pursue this principle to the point at which life had become empty of any real content. It was irrelevant to make comparisons with very disabled people who could derive satisfaction from living, because *Bland* had no life at all. In allowing him to die we would show more respect to him than by keeping him alive. He was, however, unhappy that the justification for such a decision should be that it accorded with good medical practice. Medical ethics should be formed by the law rather than the other way round. Courts should decide about a patient's best interests, which were not a matter for medical expertise. This difference of emphasis from his two colleagues and the judge of first instance was not, however, recorded as a dissenting opinion. His last point was to note that the Trust in this case had requested that a decision be reached on the assumption that its resources were unlimited. He considered that in a future case another health authority might conclude that its resources were better devoted to other patients more likely to benefit.

The Official Solicitor appealed this decision to the House of Lords where five judges unanimously rejected the appeal in February 1993. Again each wrote opinions which differed in the stress laid on different aspects of the arguments behind their concurring positions (summarized at p. 151).

Lord Keith considered that, for *Bland* himself, it was a matter of complete indifference whether he lived or died, so that comparisons with the value judgements made in other cases about the consequences of medical treatment for sensate beings were irrelevant. Doctors had no duty to continue treatment which a responsible body of medical opinion considered of no benefit (the Bolam test) (3). To emphasize this, he went on to state that deciding that there was no benefit was a matter for doctors. However, he agreed that for the time being the endorsement of the court should be sought before discontinuing treatment.

Lord Goff commented on the difficult mix of civil and criminal law that this case presented. He considered it deplorable that no guidance could be given to the medical profession, and referring to the *Barber* case in California he declared that a murder prosecution was a poor way to design a code for the behaviour of doctors. The law should provide a means of removing the obligation of a doctor to prolong life regardless of its leading to adverse and cruel effects in order to protect the self-determination of the incompetent patient. He also thought that no weighing of burdens and benefits was relevant because it was clear that treatment had no therapeutic purpose of any kind. There was therefore no duty to provide such treatment. If the justification for providing treatment for incompetent patients was that it was in their best interests, it followed that it should be discontinued if no longer in their best interests. Referring to previous cases in other jurisdictions, he noted that there was now in the course of development and acceptance throughout the common law world a community of view on the legal aspects of discontinuing treatment. He regarded doctors as competent to decide about best interests in accordance with widely accepted medical opinion. As evidence of this in the present case he quoted the BMA document and its safeguards – adequate initial treatment, waiting for 1 year, second opinions and consulting the family. However, it was doctors not the family whose opinion was determinative. Any reluctance of an individual doctor to withdraw treatment on a matter of conscience could be dealt with by a change of doctor. As for future cases he hoped that it would soon be possible to relax the present requirement for judicial review of each case, limiting court applications to cases where there were problems.

Lord Lowry declared that there was no legal distinction between omission of treatment and later withdrawing it. He hoped that *parens patriae* powers would soon be restored to the court when dealing with incompetent adults in these circumstances, or an alternative evolved through legislation by Parliament. A doctor would be acting unlawfully if he continued treatment that he believed was not in that patient's best interest.

Lord Brown-Wilkinson also believed that it needed a democratic parliamentary view on how to update the law to meet the needs of medical advances rather than relying on judge-made modifications of existing law. There were variations in the moral stance taken by professionals and the public on matters such as this. It was to the great advantage of society that doctors had hitherto exercised their own discretion in dealing with such matters. However, in hospitals there were now some staff who were so concerned with the sanctity of life that they might report doctors who took such decisions, hence the need for courts to make a declaration to protect doctors. It would be good to restore *parens patriae* for adults. He noted that the timing of a patient's death might have an impact on the rights of other parties. His pension would no longer be paid and damages recovered after a road accident or medical negligence would be much lower after death than for survival in a vegetative state. He considered that the contrast often referred to between an omission and an act was based on a distinction without a difference. Yet where, he asked, was the rationality in declaring it lawful to allow a patient to die slowly from lack of ANH but unlawful to produce the same outcome by lethal injection? It was not a question of whether it was in *Bland*'s best interest to die, rather whether it was in his best interests to continue with nonbeneficial treatment. But the whole purpose of stopping artificial feeding was to bring about the death of *Anthony Bland*. What was clear was that unless care was in a patient's best interests it must cease because the doctor was neither entitled nor under a duty to provide such care. Applying the Bolam test the BMA document provided the medical authority to withdraw treatment. The court's only concern was to be satisfied that the doctor's decision really was in accordance with accepted medical opinion. None the less, he thought doctors would be well advised to seek a legal declaration in each case. Courts may, in future, be faced with less extreme cases, such as where there was very slight sensate awareness. He stressed that his decision did not cover such a case and that he expressed no view as to what should be the answer in such circumstances.

Lord Mustill wrote the longest opinion, which began by expressing the acute unease that he felt at adopting this way through this legal and ethical maze. In dismissing this appeal, he feared that their Lordships might only emphasize the need for distortions of a legal structure which was already both morally and intellectually misshapen. The question was whether they were being asked to authorize what would otherwise be murder. The law had been left behind by new technological developments in medicine and the situation cried out for exploration by Parliament to develop new rules and procedures to protect the best interests of the community as a whole. At present doctors can proceed to treat incompetent patients in their best interests by the doctrine of necessity. This most often applied to saving life in emergency situations but, in declaring the sterilization of a mentally handicapped adult as lawful on grounds of necessity (*Re F*) an English court had extended this to a nonurgent, non-life-saving situation (4). But *Bland* had no interests of any kind and it was stretching personal rights to breaking point to say that he had an interest in ending the distress of others or in diminishing indignity. The argument that was most logically defensible within the existing law was to maintain that treatment was no longer of benefit because it could no longer serve to maintain the combination of manifold characteristics that we call a personality. There was, therefore, no duty to provide the treatment, and its omission was therefore not criminal. He had reservations about applying the Bolam principle because the decision was ethical and not medical. There was no reason in logic why the opinions of doctors should be decisive. He noted that a court would not necessarily reach the same conclusion in less extreme cases where a glimmering of awareness might give the patient an interest. He ended his opinion by stating that he felt profound misgivings about almost every aspect of this case.

The withdrawal of tube feeding was proceeded with, in spite of some local protests from pro-life groups, and *Bland* died peacefully. A Roman Catholic priest from Scotland, a zealous antiabortion campaigner, threatened a private prosecution of the doctors for murder, but the Roman Catholic bishop in whose diocese *Bland* had died advised him to desist. Since then *Bland*'s father has several times responded to journalists' questions indicating that he remains convinced that the right decision was made to let his son die.

REFERENCES

1 *In re C (A minor. Wardship: medical treatment) [1990] Fam. 26*
2 *In re J (A minor. Wardship: medical treatment) [1991] Fam. 33*
3 *Bolam* v. *Friern Hospital Management Committee* [1957] 1 W.L.R. 582
4 *In re F (Mental patient; sterilisation)* [1990] 2 A.C. 1
   For commentaries on the *Bland* decision see p. 152 and p. 165

Case of Ward of Court

Re a Ward of Court [1995] 2 ILRM 401 (Ir. Sup. Ct.)

When aged 22, this woman suffered cardiac arrest during anaesthesia for minor gynaecological surgery as a private patient in the Republic of Ireland. She was left vegetative and was sent to the National Medical Rehabilitation Centre. A claim for medical negligence was settled in court and this included care for the rest of her life in this centre, which was run by the same order of nuns as the original treating hospital. She stayed there for the next 22 years but the family, themselves Catholics, were very unhappy that the doctors and nurses never adequately discussed her condition and their treatment plan with them. In particular, their requests for no new interventions to sustain her life were ignored and she was given antibiotics and twice had general anaesthetics – for dental care and placing a gastrostomy tube. Late in 1992, she was transferred to a hospice where the doctors undertook to forgo any extraordinary measures to prolong her life, and in particular agreed that if her feeding tube became blocked the situation would be reassessed. This assurance was given to her brother, a consultant obstetrician in England. However, when her gastrostomy tube became disconnected in December 1993, she was transferred to hospital for re-placement under anaesthetic without reference to her mother, who was her Committee as a Ward of Court (a status conferred on her $2\frac{1}{2}$ years after she had become vegetative). Her mother was then asked by the hospital to give verbal consent to surgery on the telephone, which, after some protest, she unwillingly did. At subsequent meetings with the doctors and nuns at the hospice it was agreed that she was in a persistent vegetative state but they now seemed unwilling to accept a plan for future management that would amount to minimal comfort care. Some months later they claimed that she had now regained some cognitive function (23 years after the episode of brain damage), but no evidence of change was observed by her large family. The family indicated their intention of obtaining a court order to withdraw artificial nutrition.

On examination she showed visual tracking and some medical reports claimed that this indicated cognitive function, whilst some of her nurses claimed that they 'knew' that she recognized them. Some experts were sure she was vegetative, being similar to the cases that were later to be accepted in the English courts, although they did not satisfy all the eye signs of the Royal College of Physicians report (p. 161). The doctors involved in her care now rejected the diagnosis of vegetative state and one maintained that he never used this 'revolting term'. In any event, they were all completely opposed to withdrawing ANH which they regarded as ordinary care, and the hospice took the same view.

The case came before the High Court in May 1995, when the Committee of the Ward (the patient's mother), with the support of her large family, requested an order that ANH should cease. This was opposed by the hospice, the General Solicitor for Wards of Court who had been appointed her *guardian ad litem* and the Attorney General representing the public policy interest of the state. In a preliminary hearing the judge ruled that the evidence should be heard in camera with the judgement delivered in public but preserving anonymity. He also stated that whatever order the court might make the hospice ought not to be required to act contrary to its philosophy and code of ethics. Evidence was heard over 4 days and on the fifth day submissions from counsel for each of the four parties. They disagreed about the standard of proof that was appropriate. The family wanted the civil rule of more probable than not, the hospice wanted the criminal standard of beyond reasonable doubt, the guardian wanted clear and convincing and the Attorney General either this or the civil standard. The judge ruled that it should be no higher than clear and convincing because, otherwise, the court might not be able to reach a decision.

The judgement began with several pages of extracts from the *Bland* courts. The judge then stated that he was satisfied that although the *Ward* was not fully PVS such cognitive capacity as she possessed was extremely minimal. He went on to comment that, if her minimal cognition included any inkling of her catastrophic condition, that would be a terrible torment and worse than if she were fully PVS. He noted that there was a difference of opinion between some of the doctors about her condition, and between some of the Roman Catholic theologians giving evidence about what was ethical. However, it was the lawfulness not the morality of the proposed course of action that the court had to decide. Counsel for the family relied on an article of the Constitution that the family had the right to decide what was in the best interests of this patient. Whilst not doubting the *bona fides* of this family, the judge ruled that as she was a Ward of Court it was not for the family or the carers to decide but for the court to do so under its *parens patriae* jurisdiction. He observed that the State's interest in the preservation of life, as stated in the Irish Constitution, was not absolute and that a patient had a right to be allowed to die in accordance with nature. This arose from the right of autonomy, self-determination and privacy – which allowed refusal of life-sustaining treatment by competent patients. Some medical witnesses argued that this should be limited to the terminally ill (likely to survive no more than 6 months), but another observed that the *Ward* would indeed be terminally ill if life had not been artificially maintained.

The judge then spoke in general terms about withholding or withdrawing life-support systems from a terminally ill incompetent patient. He ruled that it would be proper and lawful practice to do so if the carers and surrogates agreed that this would be in the best interests of the patient. If the surrogates disagreed with the professional carers' wish to stop treatment, a second medical opinion should be obtained, and action then taken in accordance with that medical opinion. Only if the surrogates wished to stop treatment and the carers disagreed (as in the present case) should the High Court be involved.

In regard to ANH, he did not see how a method that was manifestly artificial at the outset could become normal or ordinary simply because it had continued for a long time. It was clearly a form of medical treatment and no different from a ventilator. Quoting from the *Bland* and the New Zealand case he considered that the matter turned on whether it was in the *Ward*'s best interest to have her life prolonged. In view of the clear and convincing evidence of the family, he thought it highly probable that, if the *Ward* were granted a momentary lucid period, she would choose to refuse the continuance of the present regime.

The benefit to the *Ward* of sustaining her life by artificial means of nourishment was far outweighed by the burdens of sustaining life with absolutely no prospect of any improvement. He ruled that all artificial nourishment should be terminated, and he consented to the nontreatment of infections or other pathological conditions. In the light of his earlier comments about the hospice, he authorized the family to arrange the *Ward*'s transfer to an institution willing to proceed in accordance with order of the court.

The case was appealed and heard in the Supreme Court by the Chief Justice and four other judges. The main grounds for appeal were that the order failed to vindicate the life of the *Ward* and to vindicate the right to be fed (a basic and fundamental right), and that the finding of the trial judge had been based on assessment of quality of life and this should not have been made for a person with even minimal cognition. All of these were claimed to be impermissible under the provisions of the Constitution. It was an error in law, they claimed, to have applied the test of best interests and to have applied a principle more appropriate to a terminally ill patient. The judge had misdirected himself in fact and in law by holding that ANH was medical treatment, and the standard of proof should have been beyond reasonable doubt. Some appellants had claimed that relying on *Bland* had been wrong because the presence of even minimal cognitive capacity (denied by some of the medical experts) had made the case completely different from *Bland*.

After a 5-day hearing, the appeal was dismissed 3 months after the original judgement by a four to one majority. The Chief Justice agreed that the right to life took precedence over other rights save in exceptional circumstances and that a court could never sanction steps to terminate life. Indeed, this aspect of law applied with even greater force in this jurisdiction. However, dying was a consequence of life and there was therefore a right to a natural death that was not artificially prolonged. The rights to individual privacy, to bodily integrity and self-determination were un-enumerated personal rights recognized by the Constitution and identified by previous courts. He considered that she should be regarded as terminally ill and that ANH was medical treatment that could lawfully be withdrawn. She should not be deprived of the opportunity to have someone exercise on her behalf the right of other citizens to request the lawful withdrawal of treatment, because the Constitution required that all citizens be equal before the law. Neither the common good nor public order nor morality required that the exercise of this constitutional right of the *Ward* should be restricted. As for cognitive function, he quoted at length from the trial judge's assessment of the *Ward*'s condition and ruled that, as this had been based on credible testimony, it was binding on the Appeal Court. He concluded that the trial judge had had due regard for the Constitutional rights of the *Ward*, the family and the state. Best interests had been the proper test, properly approached as they would be from the standpoint of a prudent, good and loving parent.

Another appeal judge observed that the trial judge had not blindly followed *Bland* but had applied the best interests test recommended in that case to the particular case of the *Ward*. Another judge observed that the *Ward* was not living a life in any meaningful sense and this was quite different from a severely mentally or physically handicapped person. The dissenting judgement was also the shortest. He considered that cognition had to be either present or absent and that any attempt to measure its value would be dangerous. He appeared to concede, however, that even with minimal cognitive function the court might properly have consented to withdrawal of treatment, if this had been shown to be painful and burdensome. However, he contended that tube feeding could not be so described, nor could the *Ward* be regarded as terminally ill.

What followed was described in a newspaper article by the *Ward*'s mother several months later (Irish Times 24 February 1996, p. 10). Immediately after the Supreme Court's decision there had been no difficulty in finding a nursing home, nurses and doctors willing to carry out the order of the court. However, a few days later the Irish Medical Council issued a statement that it would not be changing its existing guidance on ethical conduct in the light of the Supreme Court's decision, and asserting that ANH was a basic human need. The implication was that any doctor complying with the court order would risk disciplinary proceedings. Two weeks later, the Nursing Board of Ireland issued a statement that a nurse was not allowed to participate in the withdrawal of ANH. The doctors, nurses and nursing home who had initially been willing to help the family all retreated for fear of censure. During the next month, the family scoured the country for people willing to help, but to no avail. Meanwhile, the hospice sent a series of letters to the family requesting the urgent removal of the *Ward*. Eventually an Irish doctor and eight nurses volunteered to help and she was taken to the family home where she died peacefully 8 days after withdrawing ANH and almost 2 months after the court order. No further comment was heard from the professional organizations.

Epilogue

In the 30 years since the vegetative state was defined and named there has been a gradual evolution of medical knowledge about its diagnosis, prognosis and pathology. However, there remains much that we do not yet know – in particular about the nature of consciousness and about how even partial recovery can occur after many months. The diagnosis and prognosis remain matters of probability rather than of certainty. This makes the condition no different from many others in medicine that require decisions to be made about management in order to provide compassionate care. The medical uncertainties about the vegetative state have recently been reviewed by an English neurologist (1) who emphasized also the persisting ethical uncertainties. Some of these derive from the unresolved clinical problems, but there is also the question of the equitable use of scarce medical resources when it comes to indefinite life support for permanently vegetative patients. This is particularly difficult to justify when there is such a broad consensus among doctors, ethicists and lawyers that prolonging survival in this condition brings no benefit to the patient.

Lawyers, also, are still wrestling with the problems that these patients pose for them. In the South African case, the judge observed that the law was but a translation into policies of society's fundamental values (p. 205); whether discontinuing treatment for a permanently vegetative patient was considered wrongful had to be judged by the legal convictions and *boni mores* of a society. He concluded that reasonableness rather than logic dictated the formation of society's legal and moral convictions about what was right or wrong. In the New Zealand case, the judge considered that the issue of treatment withdrawal in these circumstances was essentially a medical one that could not be resolved by strict logic and certainly not by legal logic. It was best determined, he thought, by common principles of humanity and common sense (pp. 206–7).

Although a consensus has emerged in several jurisdictions that treatment withdrawal from these patients is lawful, many lawyers remain unhappy. They are concerned at how deviously the current law on homicide has to be reinterpreted to allow a decision to be made that most agree to be reasonable. Advances in medical technology have produced new situations that could not have been envisaged when writing the laws that still apply, and these lawyers have called for legislation to recognize this (pp. 167–8). However, there has been reluctance on the part of legislators to respond, as there was also when statutes to deal with brain death and with advance directives were considered. It may be that the view will eventually prevail in Britain, as it already does in many other places, that decision making about these patients should revert to doctors. Even without a statute, they should be reassured that the common law protects them, since so many judges have ruled that treatment withdrawal is a reasonable course of action, given adequate safeguards. These should include confirmation of the diagnosis and prognosis by more than one doctor, consultation with the family, and perhaps some formal documentation of these procedures such as the BMA suggested in its recent guidance (p. 112).

I delayed completing this book until I felt that the most contentious issues had been resolved. The guidance from the Royal College and the BMA confirm the medical position, whilst the judicial conclusion in the English High Court that current legal practice does not infringe the Human Rights Act (p. 162) has stabilized the situation for lawyers. There will doubtless continue to be some arguments and there are likely to be further developments in the medical field. None the less it seemed reasonable now to review the history so far and to take stock of the present situation.

REFERENCES

1 Wade DT. Ethical issues in diagnosis and management of patients in the permanent vegetative state. *BMJ* 2001; 322: 352–4

Index

acts and omissions   107, 114, 140, 163–4, 189, 212
advance directives   80, 120, 131, 138–9 , 141, 143, 154, 156, 157, 165, 178, 179, 182, 199, 200, 201, 202, 204
age distribution of VS   39–42
akinetic mutism   3
ALERT group   117, 164
alternative names for VS   4–5
American Academy of Neurology (AAN) 7–8, 18, 58–9, 93
American Association of Retarded Citizens 111, 199
American Geriatric Society   80, 111, 199
American Medical Association (AMA)   8, 13, 18, 35, 36, 59, 75, 106, 202
American Neurological Association (ANA) 7, 11, 13, 17, 18, 19
Americans with Disabilities Act (1990)   133
apallic syndrome   1, 51
Appleton Conference   79, 101, 104
artificial nutrition and hydration (ANH)
  alternative methods   18, 88, 110
  burdens of   112, 195, 199
  disproportionate treatment   105
  in non-PVS patients   111–12
  medical treatment or basic care   109, 112, 151, 154, 156, 191–2, 195–6, 202, 208–10, 216
  withdrawal   92–4, 128–34, 177
    difficulties in US nursing homes   141
    for conscious paralysed patients   93
    institutional refusal to comply   106, 140–2, 189
    management of   92–4
    Sloganism of starvation   93, 195
    special ethical problems   108–12
    symbolism of feeding   94, 110, 205
attitudes to minimally conscious state   82–4, 142–4
attitudes to PVS, of

AMA   75
American Geriatric Society   80, 111, 199
American pediatricians   74
Anglican Bishop of Durham   73
Appleton Conference   79, 101, 104
bioethics consultants   78
BMA   75
Cambridge physicist   73
ethicists who regard PVS patients as dead 81
European doctors   78–9, 83, 92, 176
family members   80–1, 106, 137–8
Institute of Medical Ethics   76
Japanese doctors   79
Japanese public   79
judges in *Bland*   76, 211
Justice Brennan in *Cruzan*   75
Lancet   115, 152–3,
medical students vs experts   74
President's Commission   74–5
UK doctors   78
UK press   74
US bioethicists   78
US patients and public   76–7
US physicians and nurses   77–8
see also Roman Catholic Church
Australia   183–5
autonomy
  conflict with futility   105
  ethical basis   99–101
  legal right   129–32
  of incompetent patient   101, 130–2, 211
  of physician or institution   99–100
  religious objections to   100–1
awareness   10–11, 14–18, 22, 83, 151, 161–2, 206, 213

Barber, court case   108, 136, 140, 190–2
Belgium   118, 182
beneficence   101

best interests   76, 102, 115, 132–3, 148–9,
      156–8, 167, 174, 192–3, 197, 201, 205,
      208, 210–13, 216–18
Bland (Airedale NHS Trust)   76, 147–5,
      207–14
   court cases since   157–65
   delayed reactions to court decision   165–8
   European doctors' attitudes to   176
   immediate reactions to court decision
      152–3
blinking to menace   11–12
BMA
   discussion paper on PVS   76, 116, 148–9
   Euthanasia Report   75–6, 116, 149
   guidance for withdrawing/withholding
      treatment   112, 116, 154
body weight   88
Bolam test   149, 163, 184, 211, 213
brain damage
   after head injury   50–2
   after nontraumatic acute insults   53
brain death   14, 81, 98
brain-stem reflexes   17–18, 25
brain weight   53
Brophy, court case   108, 111, 194–6

Californian study   7, 10, 18, 42, 68
Canada   183
cardiopulmonary resuscitation (CPR)   90,
      105–6, 109
Cardozo, Judge   129
cause of death *see* death
causes of VS   42–8
   acute damage   42–4
   in children   45–8, 46, 47
   in nursing home series   42
   nonacute (chronic) conditions   44, 45
   nontraumatic acute insults   40
   trauma   42–4
cerebral blood flow (CBF)   26
Child Neurology Society   9, 19, 35, 42, 45–6
children
   causes of PVS   46–7
   diagnosis of VS in infants   48
   different ages   39–42
   estimates of prevalence of VS   36
   prognosis for recovery   60–2
   prognosis for survival   68
Clarke, court case   173, 204–5
coma definition   2
coma arousal programme   90
Conroy, court case   108, 132, 137, 144,
      192–4
consent   129

cortical activity, evidence of
   complex behaviours   17–19
   electrical   25
   metabolic   17
   nystagmus   14
   visual tracking   13, 161–2
costs   102–3, 199
   see also resources
court cases in Britain
   Bland (Airedale NHS Trust)   76, 147–53,
      207–14
   Dr Cox   116
   Frenchay NHS Trust v *S*   158
   Law Hospital NHS Trust v *Lord Advocate
      and others*   168
   NHS Trusts v *Mrs M and Mrs H*   163
   Re C (baby)   160
   Re D   161
   Re G (adult patient; publicity)   159–60
   Re G (PVS)   160
   Re H (adult incompetent)   162
   Re J   205, 207
   Re M   162
   Swindon and Marlborough NHS Trust v *S*
      159
court cases in other countries
   Australia   183–5
   Canada (*Nancy B*)   173, 183, 206
   Germany (Frankfurt case)   180
   Germany (*Schwatza*)   179
   Ireland (*Ward of Court*)   175–7, 214–19
   Netherlands (*Stinissen*)   177–9
   New Zealand (*L*)   173–5, 206–7
   South Africa (*Clarke*)   173, 204–5
   Switzerland (*Widmer*)   164
court cases in US
   Baby K   133
   Barber   108, 136, 140, 190–2
   Brophy   108, 111, 194–6
   Conroy   108, 132, 137, 144, 192–4
   Cruzan   75, 111, 131, 137–9, 198–202
   Fox   112, 135
   Grant   144
   Gray   141
   Jane Doe   144
   Jobes   20, 132, 141
   Martin   143
   O'Connor   136, 137, 196–8
   Quinlan   74, 98, 112, 127–8, 135–6,
      187–90
   Rasmussen   144
   Requena   141
   Saikewicz   135
   Wanglie   106, 142

Wenland 143
Criminal law 130, 140, 147, 148, 152, 168,
    169, 179, 182, 205, 206, 208, 213
    see also murder
Cruzan, court case 75, 111, 131, 137–9,
    198–202
CT scanning 25–6

death, cause of
    after ANH withdrawal 114
    after maintained treatment 68
    legal 140, 150
decision making
    best interests 132–3
    objective judgment 132
    subjective judgment 130
    substituted judgment 131
    who decides? 132, 134–9
        courts 107, 135, 148, 150–2, 157, 165,
            168, 174, 177, 189, 192, 206, 210, 212,
            216
        family 127, 135, 137–8, 148, 160, 178,
            188–90, 192, 194, 197, 199
        physicians 136, 148, 168, 176–7, 188,
            202, 209, 211, 212
        proxies 138–9, 154, 169–70, 178, 183,
            200
        see also advance directives
decisions to abate treatment in US 1977–90
    128
definitions of VS *see* diagnosis
diagnosis
    American Academy of Neurology 8
    American Neurological Association 11
    Californian data base 7, 10
    Child Neurology Society 7, 9
    confidence in 20–3
    Higashi, Japan series 7, 8
    Japanese Neurosurgical Society 7, 8
    laboratory data 25–8
    mistaken 21–3
    Multi-Society Task Force (1994) 7, 12
    neuroimaging 25–6
    neurological findings in VS series 14–16
    Royal College of Physicians 13
dictionary definition of vegetative 4
diffuse axonal injury (DAI) 51–3
Do Not Resuscitate (DNR) order 91
Doe, Jane, court case, 144
drugs in treatment 90
duration of VS
    for definition of diagnosis 28
    for definition of permanence 61, 118, 149,
        155

for expectation of life 67
for prognosis for recovery 58, 62–3
influence on estimates of prevalence 33

electroencephalogram (EEG) 25
emotional behaviours 16
epidemiology 33–49
epilepsy 17, 162
ethics
    acts and omissions 107, 114, 140, 163–4,
        189, 212
    autonomy 99–101, 129–32
    beneficence 101
    in Belgium 118, 182
    in Britain/UK 115–18
    in France 119
    futility 105–7
    in Germany 119
    House of Lords Select Committee Report
        153–5
    international variations 115–21
    in Italy 120
    justice 102
    killing vs letting die 113–15
    maleficence 99, 101
    in Netherlands 118
    in New Zealand 120–1
    intention 108, 114, 168
    ordinary vs extraordinary treatment
        104–5, 188, 195
    principles 99–104
    sanctity of life 104
    in Scandinavia 118
    in Southern Europe 120
    special problems of ANH 108–12, 147,
        176–7
    in US 99–105
    withholding vs withdrawing 107–8
    see also Roman Catholic Church
European survey of physicians 62, 78–9, 91,
    109, 176–7
euthanasia
    ALERT group 117, 164
    BMA report 75–6, 116, 149
    ethical and legal aspects 80, 92, 103, 113,
        116, 140, 143, 151, 152, 153, 164, 166,
        167, 179, 188, 195–6, 204, 209
    House of Lords Select Committee 153–4
evidence of patient's prior wishes 193,
    194–5, 197, 198–201, 203
    see also advance directives
expectation of life *see* prognosis for survival
extraordinary vs ordinary treatment 104–5
eye movements 11–14, 161–2

family
 burdens on 101
 benefits to v patient benefits 101, 110
 see also decision-making
Fox, court case 112, 135
France 40–1, 59, 119, 181
futility 105–7, 184

Germany
 ethics 119, 180
 Frankfurt case 180
 Schwatza 179
Glasgow Outcome Scale 3, 36
Grant, court case 144
Gray, court case 141
Greece 120

head injury
 as proportion of acute causes 40–4
 incidence of VS at intervals after 37–41
 see also brain damage; prognosis for
  recovery
Higashi 8–9, 13–16
historical aspects 1–5
House of Lords
 judgements in *Bland* 151–2, 165, 210–14
 Lancet, comment on 153
 Select Committee Report 153–4
Human Rights Act (1998) 162–4

incidence studies 36–41
 incidence of acute VS in UK, USA and
  France 40–1
Institute of Medical Ethics 76, 147
institutional refusal to withdraw or continue
  treatment 106, 140–2, 189
intensive care decisions 103, 108, 113
Ireland (*Ward of Court* case) 175–7, 214–19
Italy 120

Japan
 attitudes to permanent VS 79
 definitions of VS 8
 neurological features in series 14–16
 surveys of prevalence 34, 43
Jobes, court case 132, 141
justice, as an ethical principle 102

killing vs letting die 113–15
 see also criminal law, murder

laboratory investigations 25–8
Lancet 115, 147, 152–3, 166–7
late recoveries 63–4

Law Commission
 Canada 183
 England 156–7, 162
 New Zealand 174
 Scotland 157
legal cause of death 140, 150
legal issues
 UK 147–72
 US 127–46
 other countries 173–86
 see also court cases
legislation, need for in UK 152, 154, 156,
  167, 212
liberty
 On Liberty, John Stuart Mill 99
 right to 133
limb movements 14–16
living will *see* advance directives
locked-in syndrome 20

magnetic resonance imaging (MRI) 25–6
maleficence 101
Martin, court case 143
Medical Ethics Committee, BMA 148
medical management of PVS 87–96
medical students, attitudes to PVS 74
metabolic measures of brain function 17
Mill, John Stuart, *On Liberty* 99
minimally conscious state (MCS)
 attitudes 82–4, 142–4
 definition 23–4
 legal cases in US 143–4
mortality *see* prognosis for survival
murder 136, 140, 148, 150, 152, 153, 166,
  179, 189, 190, 191, 207, 209, 210, 211,
  213, 214 *see also* criminal law
Multi-Society Task Force 3, 7, 12–13, 17–18,
  59–64, 66–7

neocortical necrosis 3
Netherlands
 ethics 118
 Health Council Statement 118
 prevalence survey 44
 Stinissen case 177–9
neuroimaging 25–6
New Zealand 120–1, 173–5, 206–7
nursing homes
 attitudes of directors 77–8
 causes of VS cases in 43
 difficulties with withdrawing ANH 141
 prevalence surveys in US 35–6
nursing management of PVS 87–96
nystagmus 13, 17–18, 162

objective judgment   132
O'Connor, court case   136, 137, 196–8
Official Solicitor
  functions   149, 208
  Practice Notes   155–6,

pain
  absence of in assessing best interests or
      quality of life   132, 193, 210
  experience of by VS patients   15, 18–19
parens patriae powers   149, 151, 157, 168,
      175, 193, 212, 216
pathology
  after nontraumatic insult   53
  after traumatic insult   51–2
  brain weight   53
  compared to damage in severely disabled
      patients   53
  cortical damage   52–4
  DAI   51–3
  thalamic damage   53–5
Patient Self-Determination Act   136, 138, 203
percutaneous endoscopic gastrostomy
      (PEG)   88
permanence of VS, when declared by
  AAN   58–9
  AMA   59
  American physicians   61–2, 92
  BMA   76
  European doctors   62, 91
  Netherland Health Council   118
  New Zealand Medical Council   174
  Official Solicitor   155
  Royal College of Physicians   155
  Task Force   61
persistent v permanent   4
personhood   81, 104
physiotherapy   88–9
Pope Pius XII   98
positron emission tomography (PET)   27–8
President's Commission   2, 74, 81, 100, 108,
      132, 134, 195
prevalence data
  Californian data base   10, 35
  child neurologists in US   35
  France   34–5
  Japan   34
  Milwaukee nursing homes   35
  Netherlands   34
  US estimates   35–6
principles of medical ethics   99–104
privacy, right to   133, 189, 200
prognosis for recovery   57–64
  AAN   58–9

AMA   59
children v adults   60–3
data before Task Force   57–9
France study   59
late recovery   63–4
prediction of recovery   64–5
relation to duration of VS   62–3
Task Force data   59–63
Traumatic Coma Data Bank   59, 63
when confident   61–2
prognosis for survival   65, 70
  Californian studies   67–9
  cause of death   69–70
  later mortality   65–6
  mean vs median expected survival   69
  of minimally conscious   69
  one-year mortality   58, 60–2, 65–6
  prolonged survival   66–7
  Task Force data   66–7
proxies *see* decision making

quality of life
  absence of pain   132, 193, 210
  in assessing beneficence   101
  best interests   75, 129, 132, 150, 199, 200,
      208, 217
  futility   105
  v sanctity of life   80, 104, 129, 196
  'worth-the-effort' quality   106
Quinlan, court case   74, 98, 112, 127–8,
      135–6, 187–90

Rasmussen, court case   144
recovery *see* prognosis for recovery
reflex responses   12–18
refusal of treatment   76–8, 100, 129, 195, 200
relatives *see* family
remitting VS   20
Requena, court case   141
resources   102–3, 106, 151, 153, 211, 221
right to liberty and privacy   133
Roman Catholic Church
  Belgium   118
  challenge to autonomy   101
  ethical stance in UK   117, 152, 153, 166, 214
  ethical stance in US   98, 103–4, 112–13,
      141, 188–9
  Ireland   117–18, 175, 214, 216
  Pope Pius XII   98
Royal College of Physicians (RCP)   8, 13–14,
      154, 161

sanctity of life   80, 104, 150–1, 167, 183, 196,
      206, 209, 212

Scandinavia   118, 182
Scottish law   148, 157, 168–70
self-determination *see* autonomy; Patient
      Self-Determination Act
sensory stimulation   90
slippery slope argument   103, 117, 129
South Africa (*Clarke*)   173, 204–5
Southern European countries   120
Spain   120
subjective judgment   130
substituted judgment   131
suicide   130, 140, 153, 167, 196
swallowing   18

Task Force *see* Multi-Society Task Force
terminally ill   103, 113, 128, 134, 156, 216
thalamic damage   27, 52–4
Traumatic Coma Data Bank   59, 63

unconsciousness   2

ventilator (respirator)   98, 128, 129, 155, 160,

173, 188, 190–1, 206–7
visual tracking (following)   12–13, 161–2

Wanglie, court case   142
Ward of Court (Ireland)   175–7, 214–19
Wenland, court case   143
withdrawing established life-sustaining
      treatments
   as default mode for PVS   107, 133
   cause of death after   114
   countervailing interests of society   129
   for competent patients   93, 128, 129
   in intensive care   103
   reasons for allowing   128–34
   relevance of expected duration of survival
      75, 114, 134, 216
   suggested VS treatment statute   132–3
   ventilation   98, 128, 129, 155, 160, 173,
      188, 190–1, 206–7
   who decides?   134–9
withholding new interventions   76–8, 91
withholding vs withdrawing   107–8, 189, 205